Meditations & Rituals *Using Aromatherapy Oils*

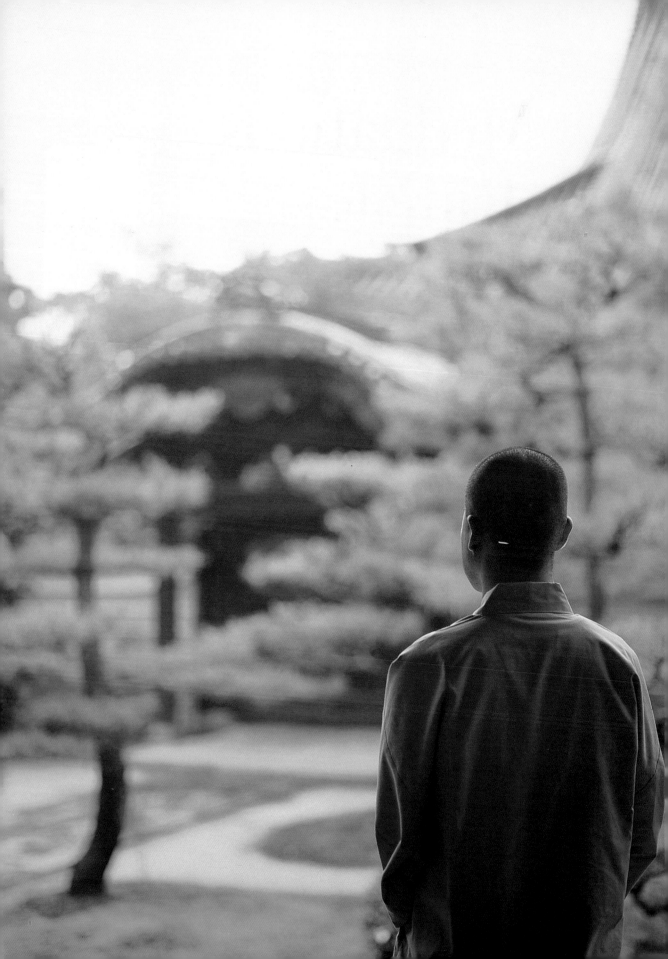

Meditations & Rituals *Using Aromatherapy Oils*

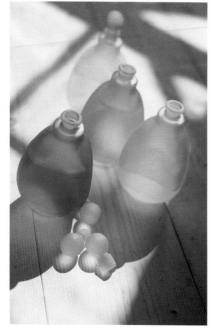

Gill
Farrer-Halls

Sterling Publishing Co., Inc.
New York

For all my spiritual teachers, with deepest gratitude

I would like to thank everyone who helped with this book. In particular, I am grateful to
the people at Godsfield Press and The Bridgewater Book Company, Lynda Marshall the
picture researcher, my excellent agent Liz Puttick, and my partner Robert Beer for his love
and support. Special thanks to Zara Elrington, Chantek Mottershaw and Lotte Rose,
dear friends on the path of aromatherapy, whose wisdom, love and strength over the
years has been invaluable.

Library of Congress Cataloging-in-Publication Data Available

10 9 8 7 6 5 4 3 2 1

Published in 2001 by Sterling Publishing Company, Inc.
387 Park Avenue South, New York, N.Y. 10016
© 2001 Godsfield Press
Text © 2001 Gill Farrer-Halls
Gill Farrer-Halls asserts the moral right to be identified as the author of this work.

Distributed in Canada by Sterling Publishing
c/o Canadian Manda Group, One Atlantic Avenue, Suite 105
Toronto, Ontario, Canada M6K 3E7
Distributed in Australia by Capricorn Link (Australia) Pty Ltd
P O. Box 6651, Baulkham Hills, Business Centre, NSW 2153, Australia

Printed and bound in China
ISBN 0-8069-2652-X

Designed by **The Bridgewater Book Company**
Picture research **Lynda Marshall**
Photography **Mike Hemsley, Walter Gardiner Photography**
Page layout **Sara Kidd**
Properties and styling **Jane Henderson**
Model **Katharine Newton**

The publishers wish to thank the following for the use of pictures:
A–Z Botanical Collection, pp. 31, 33, 38, 39, 41, 42, 45, 49, 50, 52, 76, 77, 90;
Bridgeman Art Library, p.17, San Apollonia, Ravenna;
Garden Picture Library, pp. 13, 22, 25, 26, 27, 28, 29, 34, 36, 43,
46, 47, 48, 74, 78, 86, 89, 108, 120;
Getty One Stone, pp. 2, 10, 20, 61, 63, 65, 84, 94, 102, 104, 106, 114, 115, 122;
Harry Smith Collection, pp. 16, 19, 30, 32, 37, 40, 44, 51, 53;
Hutchison Library, pp. 9, 24.
Image Bank, pp. 6, 7, 14, 23, 58, 60, 64, 80, 82, 92, 96, 98, 99, 100, 110, 111, 112, 118.

The publishers wish to thank the following for help with properties:
Antique Interiors, Bright Ideas, Spellbound and Spirit,
The Elephant's Trunk, Tizz's, all located in Lewes, East Sussex.

CONTENTS

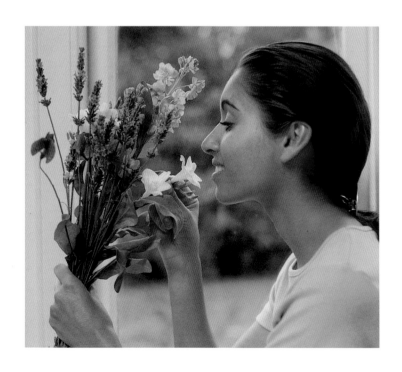

Aromatherapy and Essential Oils

> *"There are many ways to bring ritual and self-awareness into your life and essential oils are an excellent tool to use."*
>
> **JANINE MURPHY:** *AROMATHERAPY TODAY*

TODAY THE TERM "AROMATHERAPY" IS WELL-known, and aromatherapy practice is established in many countries. Yet when I trained in this art of esoteric healing just over a decade ago, I remember many people were unfamiliar with the word, a common response being "aroma what?"!

As well as professional aromatherapists working with essential oils mainly through massage, many people also use essential oils at home. They are a wonderful addition to the first-aid cupboard and also enhance the effects of normal skin care and beauty products. The more adventurous among us also try essential oils in the bath and vaporizers or burners, and we might intuit that there are other dimensions in which we can use these precious oils.

Historically, aromatic plants were used as aids to meditation and in rituals and ceremonies. Contemporary science reveals how essential oils work on the different areas of our brain and affect our mood and how we think, as well as healing our bodies. So we can certainly learn how to work with essential oils in the spiritual side of our lives too.

Consciousness and emotions

The right side of the brain is concerned with intuitive thought and behavior; the left side deals with more logical and intellectual processes. Feelings of calm and well-being are produced in the individual when the two sides are in harmony, an effect that can be produced by essential oils.

We have probably all had a strongly nostalgic experience caused by a sudden whiff of something familiar. Perhaps the scent of lavender bushes in a summer garden reminds us of a happy childhood, or we smell the sea and are reminded of a seaside vacation. Why should our sense of smell be such a powerful trigger?

Most of our senses are transmitted through our central nervous system, but the olfactory nerves are

Seaside memories

The smell of the ocean can evoke memories of a summer vacation. The sight of fireweed with its distinctive purple flowers is a common sight near the seaside.

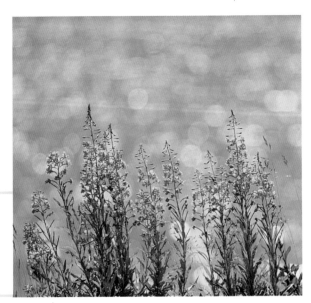

situated at the top of the nose and connect to the brain directly. Nerves link the area of the brain where smell is registered, called the limbic area, to the hypo-thalamus, which helps regulate the secretion of hormones and the autonomic nervous system. In this way, smell strongly affects our unconscious and vital functions such as hunger and sexuality. Sniffing out the next meal, a sexual partner, or an enemy were basic survival strategies for primitive humankind. Indeed, "the sense of smell is very closely linked to the proverbial 'sixth sense'" (Robert Tisserand: *Aromatherapy for Everyone*).

As civilization progressed our sense of smell became less important, but we are still attracted by "good" smells and repelled by "bad" smells—which, for example, helps us to avoid poisoning ourselves by eating food that has gone bad. Essential oils affect our moods and emotions, as part of our physiology. Combining essential oils with meditation and ritual therefore has huge potential. If we are sad, the uplifting

> *"Some experiments done with volunteers showed that when they inhaled essential oils the activity of the two sides of the brain came into closer symmetry with each other."*
>
> **PATRICIA DAVIES:**
> **AROMATHERAPY: AN A–Z**

scent of an antidepressant oil will cheer the mood and relax the body. If we perform some ritual or meditate at the same time, the effects are immeasurably increased.

Meditation and ritual

Meditation is another subject that has become more familiar in recent years. The Eastern religions of Buddhism, Hinduism, and Islam are becoming more common in Europe and the United States as the modern world dissolves old East–West boundaries. This has sparked a corresponding interest in our own spiritual traditions, particularly the contemplative aspects of Christianity and Judaism, as well as the search to rediscover our Pagan heritage.

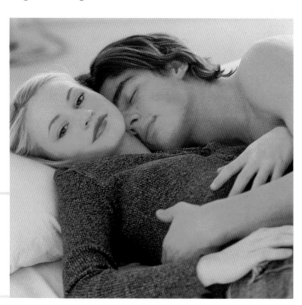

Sexual chemistry

Although we no longer find our sexual partners by smell, we are unconsciously attracted to each other by our body odors, and we enjoy the smell of our loved one.

In the old Celtic and Nature religions we find many rituals and ceremonies—such as the sorcerer's journey using aromatic herbs in the ancient Saxon *Way of Wyrd*: "We can, with the help of spearwort, project your shadow-soul from your body like a luminous personal spirit. Then you will be able to journey to the Underworld." Here the sorcerer is instructing his apprentice how to travel on the astral plane by inducing a trancelike state using spearwort.

Much ancient knowledge was lost, as civilization evolved. Yet some traditional cultures still offer living examples of religious and secular rituals. Sufi whirling dervishes (Muslim mystics), Hindu saddhus (holy men), and Tibetan lamas (Buddhist teachers), for example, still perform ancient spiritual practices.

Spiritual wisdom and essential oils

We can see how the esoteric riches of the past still live on in the present, if we are willing to seek them out, and we can experience their power and wisdom for ourselves. Reading about such subjects is interesting, but it is only by practicing meditation and ritual with essential oils that we can truly understand these ancient traditions. So this book is practical, with instructions and advice on how to meditate and perform rituals, as well as giving relevant background information.

The book creates an alchemical "marriage" between meditation and ritual with essential oils. It brings together ancient spiritual wisdom with a modern way of using aromatic plants—the distillation

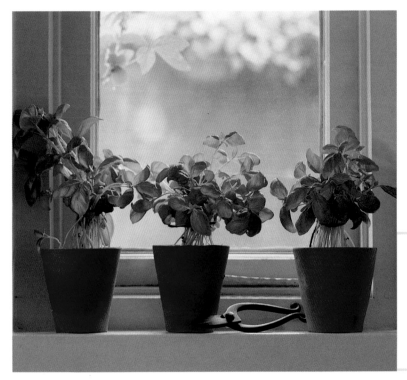

Basil
Basil is a common sight on many kitchen windowsills because it is used in cooking. The fresh, stimulating smell of basil is also useful in some meditations and rituals.

Temple offering

This man is offering lotus flowers during a religious ceremony called a *puja* in India. Huge quantities of different flowers are offered every day.

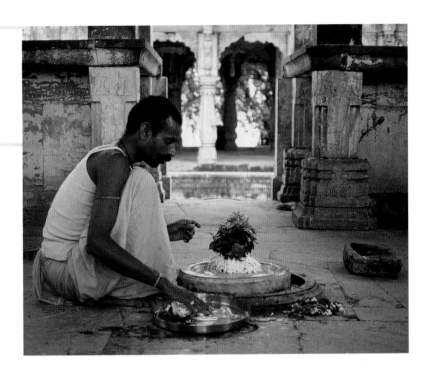

of essential oils. The practices suggested are therefore relevant for us today, and it is perhaps unsurprising that essential oils are simpler to use than aromatic plants in their natural state. As with so much else in our modern world, we have found the easy way, though this makes these meditations and rituals no less valuable, simply more accessible.

Once you have practiced the various meditations and rituals and have learned what is necessary in each case, you can create your own to reflect your individual needs and desires. Various blends of essential oils are suggested, but again listening to your intuition and what your sense of smell tells you will help you find personal blends that really work for you, alongside individual essential oils that hold special meaning.

The reader is thus invited on a journey of inner discovery. But, as with all spiritual journeys, each person must discover for himself or herself which meditations, rituals, and essential oils work at which times and for which moods.

There are instructions for simple yet powerful meditations and rituals, and descriptions of the spiritual characteristics of many well-known essential oils together with suggested blends. This will help you choose those that are appropriate in different circumstances.

However, you must find your own way to unlock the spiritual potential inside you, by trying things out, not just by reading about them. In this way the book is a guide to help you discover your own path to the sacred use of essential oils.

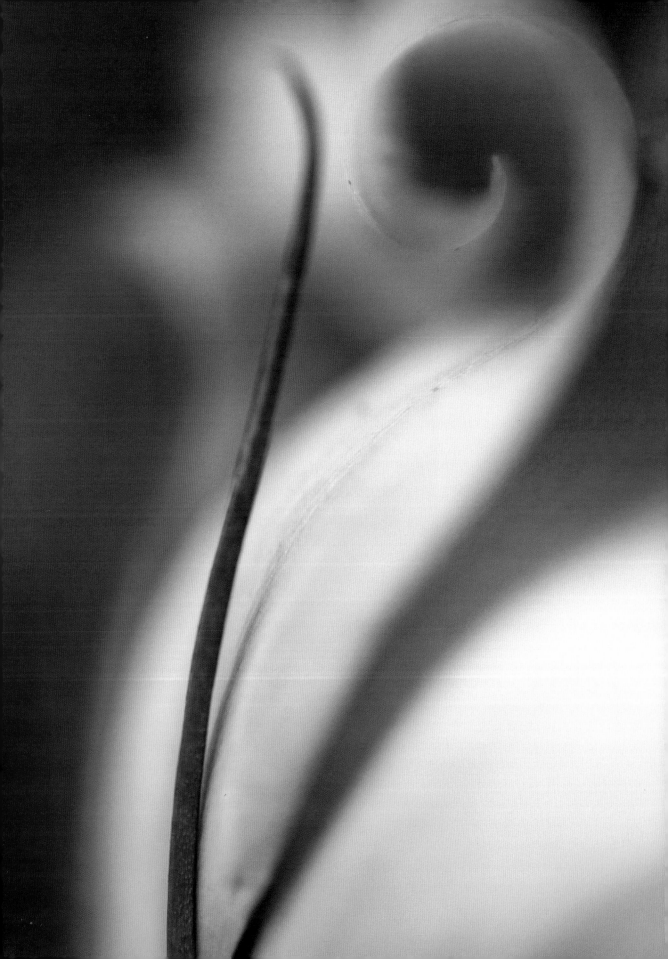

the Souls of Plants

The essence of the plant is its life energy, like the blood in our bodies. Plant essences give the plant many of its characteristics, and we could say the essence is the plant's personality. The distilled essence gives us essential oils, which are the spirit, or soul, of the plant. We must nurture these essences by treating them carefully, otherwise they will lose this precious life force, and deteriorate.

ethereal
ethereal

"The **essence** is the most ethereal and subtle part of the plant, and its therapeutic action takes place on a higher, more **subtle** level than that of the whole, organic plant, or its extract, having in general a much more pronounced effect on the mind and **emotions**."

ROBERT TISSERAND: *THE ART OF AROMATHERAPY*

subtle

What are Essential Oils?

"In their search for the philosophers' stone, elixir of life, or fountain of youth, alchemists discovered the soul of the plant— a name they gave these ethereal oils."

SUSANNE FISCHER-RIZZI:
COMPLETE AROMATHERAPY HANDBOOK

ESSENTIAL OILS ARE DERIVED FROM AROMATIC essences within plants. Essences naturally occur in some plants as part of the mystery and wonder of Nature. They help the plant thrive in various ways, such as attracting bees for pollination and repelling animals and insects. But just as we may see a flower as beautiful and a tree as magnificent, we are also inspired by sweet-scented plants.

From essence to essential oil

Aromatic essences are found within different plants and different parts of plants from around the world. Essential oils are obtained from spices, woods, resins, flowers, herbs, berries, roots, and bark. The orange tree, for example, produces three essential oils: petitgrain from the leaves and twigs, orange from the rind, and neroli from the flowers. The plant essence is transformed into its essential oil through a process of extraction (usually distillation) or, as in the case of fruit rinds, by simple expression. This is something we are familiar with; for example, when we peel a lemon we also squeeze the essence from the rind, and this tastes quite different from the juice.

Although they are called oils, essential oils are not oily; they are nongreasy, and some are as thin and light as water. However, in common with other oils, essential oils do not dissolve in water. They dissolve in base oils, also called fixed oils, such as sunflower, almond, and olive, and also in alcohol. They are highly concentrated and can be toxic if used incorrectly, but this gives them their power. They are also volatile and swiftly evaporate when exposed to air, which gives them their perfuming ability.

Aromatic plant essences have complex chemical structures based on the process of photosynthesis, which transforms the energy of sunlight and combines it with nutrients from soil, water, and air. This gives a holistic balance between the four elements of fire, earth, water, and air, and means the

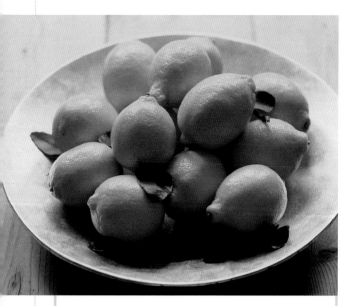

Lemons

Lemons produce both juice and essential oil. It is simple to produce a few drops of lemon essential oil by squeezing the rind, so you can use your own essential oil of lemon, if you choose.

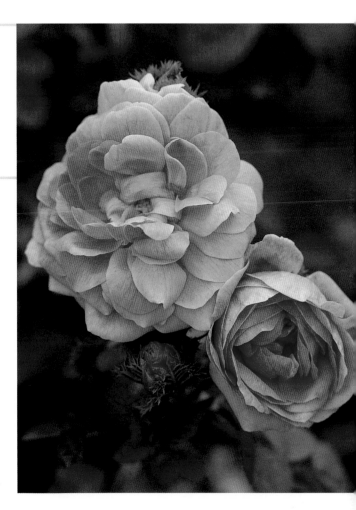

Rosa centifolia

Rosa centifolia is only one of several different types of roses used in the production of essential oil of rose. Each one has its own particular odor, and with experience we can learn to distinguish between them.

basic structure of essential oils is formed around oxygen, carbon, and hydrogen. The chemical compounds break down into two main groups: hydrocarbons and oxygenated compounds. Hydrocarbons are made up of terpenes, and oxygenated compounds of esters, aldehydes, ketones, alcohols, phenols, and oxides, though there are many trace elements as well—some as yet unclassified.

Individual characteristics

Essential oils are living organisms and continue to change subtly over time. This also means each plant that an essential oil is derived from has some unique features as well as those it shares with other plants of the same species.

No two living things are identical, though they can be very similar. This means that different batches of essential oils will be slightly, sometimes greatly, different from each other. The same is true in wine production; certain years produce finer wines than other years. Country, altitude, and soil type all affect the character of the essential oil as well. Essential oils are also derived from different subspecies of a particular plant; so, for example, there is rosa centifolia and rosa damascena, two different varieties of roses.

This means that no two bottles of rose or other essential oil will smell exactly the same. As you learn more about the oils by smelling them, you will detect more subtle levels in the different aromas, and may eventually have two or three different bottles of some essential oils because you like them for different reasons.

Historical Use of Aromatic Plants and Essential Oils

"Through burning aromatic plants they [our ancestors] would have discovered other properties; sometimes the smoke would be 'good to breathe,' sometimes it would make one feel drowsy or invigorated. 'Smoking' a patient is one of the earliest recorded forms of treatment with herbs... often used to drive out evil spirits."

ROBERT TISSERAND:
THE ART OF AROMATHERAPY

UNTIL THE DISTILLATION OF ESSENTIAL OILS was discovered—possibly by the Persian philosopher Avicenna during the tenth century, but perhaps earlier—the use of aromatic plants consisted of infused and macerated oils, pomades, and even simply crushed herbs and flowers. All these methods produce traces of essential oil, which is freed by crushing or infusing the plant.

Aromatic oils were highly prized in the ancient Egyptian, Chinese, Indian, Greek, and Roman civilizations. Originally they were used only by royalty and high priests. This was partly because the oils were expensive, but also because they were considered to be the perfumes of the gods. In later years they became more widely used, but aromatic oils never lost their original religious associations.

The Egyptian queen Cleopatra is reputed to have seduced Mark Antony not with her beauty, but with her skill with perfumes and presentation. Legend states that she sailed down the Nile to meet him with the sails of her ships impregnated with oil of rose, the most aphrodisiac of perfumes.

The ancient Indian herbal medical system, Ayurveda, which uses aromatics extensively, is still practiced today. Sandalwood is a prime ingredient, and the finest sandalwood is grown in Mysore, in central India. Sandalwood has always been a major constituent of incense and is used in a paste smeared onto the foreheads of holy men.

The medieval herbalists of Europe were well aware of the healing powers of aromatics, particularly those of native herbs such as marjoram, thyme, rosemary, and chamomile, but not exclusively. The great

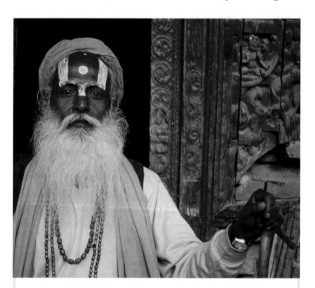

Sandalwood paste

This saddhu, or holy man, wears paste containing sandalwood, ritually applied every day as part of his devotional practice. Sandalwood paste has been used in this way for centuries.

seventeenth-century herbalist Nicholas Culpeper wrote about a wide range of aromatic plants, for both healing and cosmetic purposes. He was an astrologer and incorporated this knowledge in his writing, ascribing a ruling planet to many aromatic plants.

Medieval herbalists linked the concept of the four humors with the elements: sanguine with air, phlegmatic with water, choleric with fire, and melancholic with water. This has an interesting parallel with the Chinese technique of diagnosing illnesses according to the elements and the balance between yin and yang. Yin is female, dark, moist, and cool; yang is male, bright, dry, and hot. "Disease" was treated by restoring the balance between yin and yang; so fever (caused by an excess of yang) would be treated with cooling yin preparations. Aromatic oils were used in both healing systems to restore equilibrium; so, for example, ginger was used for its fiery yang qualities, chamomile for its cooling yin properties.

The finest frankincense was grown in southwest Arabia. This gave the country great political and economic power, because frankincense, alongside many aromatics and spices, was a major trading commodity. This was still the case in the sixteenth century when the English dramatist William Shakespeare refered to the perfumes of Arabia in his play *Macbeth*. Lady Macbeth goes mad after arranging several murders. She sleepwalks and says to herself: "Here's the smell of blood still. All the perfumes of Arabia will not sweeten this little hand."

Another reason for the famed perfumes of Arabia was the discovery (or rediscovery) of distillation in

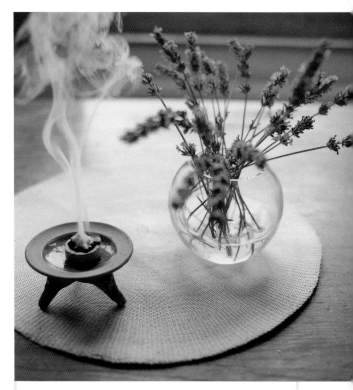

Frankincense
Here frankincense is being burned next to a vase of lavender flowers. Frankincense was a major trading commodity in ancient Arabia and is still exported from this region today.

the tenth century, thereby making pure essential oils available. Avicenna was a remarkable man who wrote almost a hundred books, as well as performing chemical and alchemical experiments. Because of the captivating scent of roses, perfumes of rose were in high demand, and Avicenna experimented to see if he could make rosewater. As a byproduct he noticed oil floating on top of the aromatic water, and so pure rose essential oil came into being.

Essential Oils in a Spiritual Context

"Indian yogis have taught for millennia that sweet-smelling aroma—in the form of [essential] oils, herbs or incense—should be used to stimulate creativity and raise the spiritual element. This is, indeed, why aroma is an integral part of religious rituals in many denominations all over the world."

VALERIE ANN WORWOOD: *AROMANTICS*

OVER THE CENTURIES PEOPLE DISCOVERED WAYS to extract plant essences so that we could use them to enrich our lives. Although plants are sacrificed to obtain their precious essences, the resulting essential oils carry the soul of the plant into another dimension, where we use them in the healing and perfuming arts. We also utilize plant essences for religious and mystical ceremonies, and this perhaps best honors their natural mystery.

Aromatics have been used since ancient times for religious and spiritual purposes. In one of the earliest archeological excavations of a grave, traces of herbs were discovered; presumably they had been part of a funerary rite. Indian and Tibetan meditations and religious rituals have used incense for thousands of years, and the principal ingredients of both Indian and Tibetan incense are aromatic plants. Catholic churches still burn frankincense during services, as they have done for centuries.

The Egyptians used aromatic compounds containing cedarwood, frankincense, sandalwood, and myrrh for embalming the dead, and the mummified body would be entombed together with pots of aromatic unguents that helped to send the spirit of the dead on its journey. The best preserved mummies

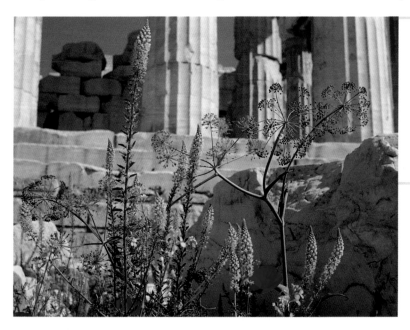

The Parthenon

Wild poppies and mignonette growing in front of the famous Greek temple, the Parthenon. When the Parthenon was still functioning as a temple, flowers would have been cultivated nearby for use in decorating the temple.

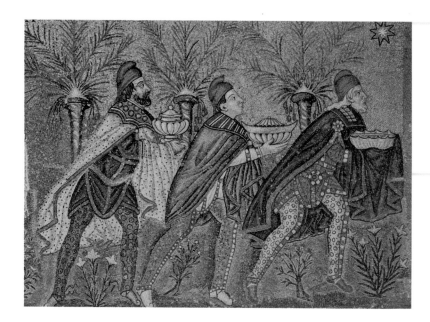

are the ones most thoroughly embalmed with a lot of oils, which has led to the modern use of these essential oils in rejuvenating skin creams!

Every culture has a vision of either paradise, the heavens, or the god realm, which looks and sounds beautiful. This idea of beauty also extends to smells. The Bible describes God and the angels entering paradise thus: "Every leaf in paradise began to sway, causing every person born of Adam to fall asleep from a wonderful fragrance." The high value—both in terms of cost and spiritual riches—ascribed to aromatics can be seen from the story of the three kings. The three most precious gifts they could offer Jesus included two aromatic gums: frankincense and myrrh.

In Egypt, at the City of the Sun, incense was burned three times a day as an offering to the Sun God, Ra. Resin (probably frankincense) was offered at dawn, myrrh at noon, and kyphi at sunset. This last was a blend containing sixteen aromatics, and according to the Greek writer Plutarch, kyphi "lulled one to sleep, allayed anxieties, and brightened dreams."

Greek mythology attributes the gods with inventing perfumes, and all aromatic plants were considered to have a divine origin. High priestesses dispensed aromatic potions at the Temple of Aphrodite to heal both the spirit and the body. The German words *heilen* (healing) and *heilig* (holy) show this connection clearly.

In sixteenth-century Europe, many essential oils—called chymical oils—were available from the apothecary to those who could afford them, and the advent of printing helped to spread information about them together with pictures of stills. This brought experimentation with the distillation of essential oils into the hands of the philosopher alchemists, who were trying to transform base metal into gold.

However, this was merely a metaphor for refining human life into its most spiritual and true nature. This religious quest for inner transformation equated the purified human psyche (which the alchemists called the quintessence) with essential oils. As essential oils evaporate into ether, burned as an offering to the gods, so does the purified human soul yearn to become one with God.

Handling Essential Oils Safely

"The present Aromatherapy recommendations commonly given are more than cautious. I sense they are creating more a mood of fear among both practitioners and public... In contrast, there are certainly negative, toxic aspects to the misuse and overdosing of essential oils."

RON GUBA: *AROMATHERAPY TODAY, VOL 11*

ESSENTIAL OILS ARE POWERFUL, AND SO highly prized that they are offered to the Divine. This reflects their precious and potent nature. It takes thousands of jasmine petals to produce a single drop of jasmine essential oil, so jasmine is expensive, and in the old days rare. This precious potency must be respected; therefore, we need to learn how to use essential oils safely and well.

Purchase and storage

Essential oils are easy to obtain. This makes them no less precious—or expensive! But it means we need to know that our essential oils have been produced, bottled, and stored correctly. Buying cheap, inferior essential oils for meditation and ritual is pointless.

Whether you get a price list from a specialist supplier or are looking in a store, you should first check that botanical names are used, for example *lavandula officinalis* rather than just lavender. There are several different species of lavender available, so it might also be called *lavandula*

angustifolia; what is important is that the supplier knows the product they are supplying.

If a range of essential oils is being offered at one price for all oils, they are not true essential oils; they will be adulterated or diluted and therefore unsuitable. You should also check the bottles. Essential oils must be stored in dark glass—brown, blue, or green—and not plastic. Essential oils are living, potent substances and chemically affect plastic. The caps and dropper inserts are plastic, but they only come into momentary contact with the essential oil as it is used.

Once you have carefully purchased your essential oils, you must store them well. It is most important to avoid direct contact with sunlight. Remember that essential oils are organically active and deteriorate quickly when exposed to extremes of heat or cold.

Essential oils have their own natural vibration and are sensitive to loud noise, pollution, and so on. Though this might sound strange, remember they are used for psychic detoxification and purification, so they are obviously very sensitive. You might like to acquire a special wooden box that keeps the individual bottles upright. These can be beautiful as well as practical and honor the precious nature of essential oils.

Safety

Essential oils are powerful and highly concentrated and can be toxic if used incorrectly. If we handle oils carefully, respecting their potency and following guidelines, they are quite safe. Never take them orally. Some essential oils can cause skin irritation if they are applied undiluted to the skin, though there will be instructions for using certain oils for perfumes and anointing.

A good general rule is not to use them neat on your skin unless you are specifically instructed to do so. Follow the instructions carefully, and never use more than suggested. Some essential oils, such as bergamot, are phototoxic; they cause skin discoloration in sunlight, so care must be taken when using them.

Avoid contact with your eyes. If you accidentally splash a drop in your eyes, do not attempt to wash them with water—essential oils do not dissolve in water—but wash them with a small quantity of base oil such as almond. This will dilute and remove the essential oil, which can be absorbed along with the base oil in a soft cloth.

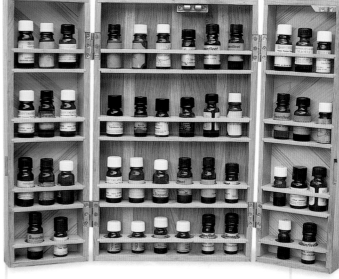

Oil box
This hand-crafted wooden box offers a beautiful and practical way to keep your essential oils safely; sunlight is avoided and the bottles are stored upright.

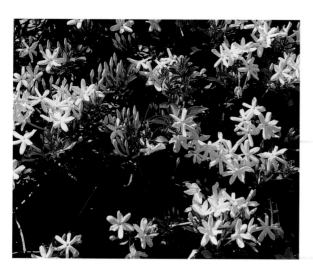

Jasmine
Jasmine essential oil, known as an absolute, is precious and expensive because it takes thousands of petals to produce a single drop. The smell strengthens at night, so the flowers are harvested at this time.

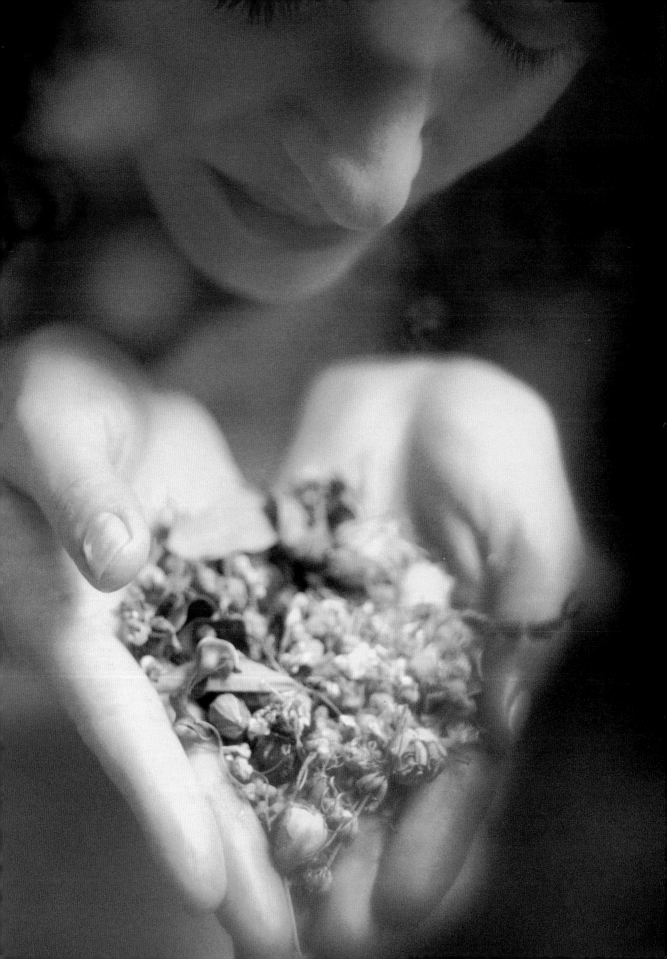

Essential Oils for Meditation and Ritual

The direct link between the olfactory nerves and the limbic system (the part of the brain that manages memory and emotion) means scents can evoke an immediate and powerful reaction that has nothing to do with our usual thought processes and that defies rational analysis. It is logical, therefore, that aromatics have consistently been used in organized religion and for personal communion with gods and spirits throughout all cultures and historical periods. The use of essential oils for meditation and ritual is merely the latest in a chain of aromatic ceremonies that humankind has used to transcend ordinary consciousness.

"There is no doubt that throughout history **aromatic** oils have been used for their **power** to influence the emotions and states of mind: this is the basis for their employment as **incense** for religious and **ritualistic** purposes."

JULIA LAWLESS: *THE ENCYCLOPEDIA OF ESSENTIAL OILS*

Roman Chamomile
Anthemis nobilis

German Chamomile
Matricaria chamomilla

CHAMOMILE IS ONE OF THE oldest recorded medical herbs. It has always been widely used in Europe but was also used by the ancient Egyptians and the Moors. Chamomile was called "maythen" by the Saxons and was one of their nine sacred herbs.

British folklore often describes chamomile's healing powers, and it was one of the "strewing herbs" of the Middle Ages. Today we walk on chamomile lawns in much the same way, releasing the fragrance as the flowers and leaves are trodden on. Chamomile is queen of the cooling, tranquil essential oils; it is ruled by Venus and is yin.

> Chamomile was called "maythen" by the Saxons and was one of their nine sacred herbs.

Chamomile is antidepressant and sedative, mirroring its calming and anti-inflammatory action on the body. Its feminine properties generally work wonderfully for premenstrual and menstrual pains, but not just the physical symptoms.

Its pronounced effect on the nervous system and the mind makes chamomile useful for meditations and rituals where there is a feeling of being hysterical or out of control. Chamomile is also useful when you are feeling "liverish" because it has a powerful tonic effect on the liver. This makes it useful for irritability, impatience, and anger—where these are flaming and hot, rather than dull or sullen.

The low toxicity of chamomile is reflected in its traditional use for children's complaints. In *A Modern Herbal*, twentieth-century herbalist Mrs. M. Grieve describes chamomile as having a wonderfully soothing, sedative, and absolutely harmless effect. We all feel childish from time to time, and chamomile soothes these peevish feelings and restlessness, without suppressing the inner child.

With its daisylike flowers, chamomile is a familiar image associated with sunny days in the countryside, and the fragrance of both Roman and German chamomiles remind us of this. The Greeks called it "kamai melon," or ground apple. The scent has hints of apple among bitter, herbaceous undertones, and warm, sweet, flowery top notes. Chamomile blends well with citrus and other floral oils. It should be avoided during the first three months of pregnancy.

Lavender

Lavandula vera

> *"Lavandula is the essence of the soul, magnetic and formative, the perfect symbol of gentleness and maternal love which mythology represented through the traits of the Mother Goddess."*
>
> **PHILIPPE MAILHEBIAU:**
> **PORTRAITS IN OILS**

LAVENDER IS THE BEST-known and most widely used of all essential oils. Neither strongly yang nor yin, its main quality is balancing. It is ruled by Mercury, the great communicator. Lavender is cultivated mainly in France, where it is also called blue magic.

Lavender has long been applied as an anointing oil, particularly on the temples, behind the ears, and on the wrists. As well as the obvious property of being a perfume, lavender helps prevent headaches, swooning, and fainting, and is known to calm turbulent emotions. Lavender water was often used to scent handkerchiefs and scarves.

The word "lavender" comes from the Latin *lavare*, which means "to wash." The Romans used lavender in their bathing water, and also for washing clothes and linen. A ritual bath with lavender helps wash away emotional and psychological debris as well as washing the body clean.

Lavender is useful in rituals and meditations to focus the mind if it swings from one thing to another. It also clears the head and is useful for indecisiveness. Culpeper advised its use for "tremblings and passions of the heart." As a heart tonic, lavender is useful if emotional pain is felt in the heart.

The clean, fresh, floral scent of lavender is sometimes linked with old ladies and lavender linen bags; it is not a modern perfume and gives a mature note to blends. This can be useful for recalling memories and childhood experiences. Avoid lavender during the first three months of pregnancy.

Frankincense

Boswellia carteri

> *"[Frankincense] has an elevating, warming, soothing effect on the mind and emotions. This recalls its traditional use in the driving away of evil spirits, if we think of these spirits rather as obsessions, fears and anxieties which may have become manifest as physical illness."*
>
> ROBERT TISSERAND:
> *AROMATHERAPY FOR EVERYONE*

WE LEARN FROM A THIRTEENTH-century French manuscript that frankincense means "luxuriant incense." It was often simply called incense and has been much used in incense since ancient times. This makes frankincense one of the most important essential oils for meditation and ritual, for it continues a long-standing tradition. Frankincense is yang, warm, and masculine; its ruling planet is the sun.

If we look at the physical properties of frankincense, we can understand its popularity in spiritual practice. Frankincense has the ability to slow down and deepen our breathing. This makes us feel calm and centered, which is how we aim to feel when we meditate. Combining frankincense with meditation therefore has the potential to increase and reinforce these feelings.

The ability to slow and deepen the breath makes frankincense useful when we are anxious, nervous, or stressed.

Anxiety makes our breathing too quick and shallow, so we don't inhale enough oxygen and, therefore, our anxiety and nervousness tend to increase. Frankincense can help to break this vicious circle and to restore balance and calm by grounding us in our body.

Frankincense is useful in rituals and ceremonies, as much today as in the past. As we see from the above quotation, with the benefit of contemporary psychological insight we can understand and name these "evil spirits" and exorcise them through ritual. What was called "possession" in ancient times is what we might call "hysteria" today, often brought about by not dealing with nervous, anxious stress and allowing it to get out of hand.

Frankincense smells divine and remains an appropriate offering to the gods. We can recall that frankincense was one of the three precious gifts offered to the baby Jesus. It combines citrus, fresh, turpentine top notes with undertones of sweet, warm, balsamic wood smoke, and blends easily, particularly with florals and woods.

Violet Leaf

Viola odorata

> Violet leaf is excellent at alleviating anxiety and is indicated for meditations and rituals that seek to allay this, and where a yin oil is preferred.

BOTH THE FLOWERS AND leaves of violets have been used extensively in herbal traditions. Violet leaf is an absolute, which means it is obtained by solvent extraction from a concrete. This makes violet leaf highly concentrated and powerful, and, like all absolutes, it should be treated with respect.

The Greeks and Romans used violets to flavor wine, believing they would prevent or cure a hangover. They were also used by the eleventh-century mystic Hildegard of Bingen to treat breast tumors, with some success. In aromatherapy, violet leaf has been used effectively for menstrual pains and irregularities, and this reflects its dark, feminine, mysterious yin nature. Violet leaf is a very calming oil and useful for insomnia.

Violet leaf is excellent at alleviating anxiety and is indicated for meditations and rituals that seek to allay this, and where a yin oil is preferred. Italian doctor Professor Paolo Rovesti uses certain essential oils, including violet leaf, to help people with psychological disturbances. He comments that: "Patients feel as if transported into a different, more agreeable and acceptable world."

The scent of violets was reputed to "comfort and strengthen the heart," which makes violet leaf a useful addition in a blend for a ritual in coming to terms with the loss of a relationship, particularly if this is recent. Violet leaf blends well with rose and complements its tonic effect on the heart.

Violet leaf has been traditionally used in the perfume industry because it not only smells wonderful but is also a good fixative. This means that violet leaf will stabilize and bring harmony to a blend, literally fixing the different aromas into one scent. It has a subtle green top note, like fresh mown hay, with elusive, heady, floral undertones. It blends beautifully with many essential oils.

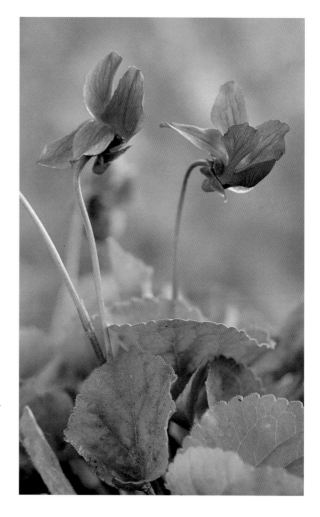

Ylang Ylang

Cananga odorata

YLANG YLANG MEANS "FLOWER of flowers," and its sweet floral smell certainly lives up to its name. The yellow flowers grow on huge trees in Madagascar, Sumatra, and Java, where local women traditionally wear the fresh flowers in their hair. Ylang ylang is a powerful aphrodisiac, and several somewhat unusual case histories are a testament to this quality!

Ylang ylang has traditionally been used to help create euphoric mind states, and modern research reveals that the scent can stimulate the release of endorphins in the brain. So ylang ylang has a potent

> *"And from the mountains and woods, flowers and high mosses, In the warm and rarefied air, released in a gust, Blows a wave of heavy sweet scents, Full of passion and sensual delights."*
>
> **LECONTE DE LISLE**

effect on the nervous system and is indicated in meditations and rituals where intensity is required; ylang ylang is not a subtle fragrance!

Ylang ylang is a useful essential oil in intimate massage between lovers, especially if there is impotence or frigidity. Its overwhelming heavy sweetness makes some men unreceptive to the smell on its own, but it blends easily, especially with light, fresh, citrus oils. Ylang ylang allows men to reveal their feminine side and enables them to become soft and receptive. It is obviously yin and is ruled by Venus.

The strength of anger and the blackness of depression meet a powerful adversary in ylang ylang. Its antidepressive, sedative qualities are reinforced by its ability to lower blood pressure, a property called "hypotensor." These qualities make ylang ylang suitable in a blend for a meditation where anger is red and hot, rather than dull and resentful, and where depression causes a lot of nervous tension, rather than lethargy.

Ylang ylang is much used in the perfume industry for its voluptuous exotic fragrance. Care must be taken not to overdo it, because too much can cause headaches, and it is perhaps best used in a blend, especially with citrus oils. Ylang ylang has been called the poor person's jasmine, because it smells similar but is considerably cheaper. The top note is intensely almond, floral sweet, with rich, creamy, almost spicy undertones.

Patchouli
Pogostemon cablin

> People who grew up in the 1960s tend to either love or hate it, and can often clearly recall incidents associated with its smell.

PATCHOULI COMES FROM INDIA and has diverse uses, such as a perfume and insect repellent for clothes, and a remedy for snakebite. However, patchouli is also grounding and its musky earthiness literally "earths" our energy.

Patchouli helped bring essential oils into popularity by being an indispensable accessory in the 1960s. Doubtless patchouli featured in the exploration of meditation and ritual that characterized this era, but evidence remains largely anecdotal. We can see the power of smell on memory strongly with patchouli; people who grew up in the 1960s tend to either love or hate it, and can often clearly recall incidents associated with its smell.

Patchouli is strongly yang and ruled by the sun. Interestingly—just like the sun—it tends to be stimulating in small doses and sedative in larger amounts. It is an excellent antidepressant and helps dispel anxiety, so is useful for a meditation or ritual for depression when you need grounding and calming. It can be an aphrodisiac—but only if both parties enjoy the scent!

The smell has been described "like old socks" as well as musky, rich, and earthy, so if you don't like it, don't use it! A little goes a long way, and the scent lingers. In small amounts patchouli gives blends an oriental flavor; it is a great fixative and blends well with other oils.

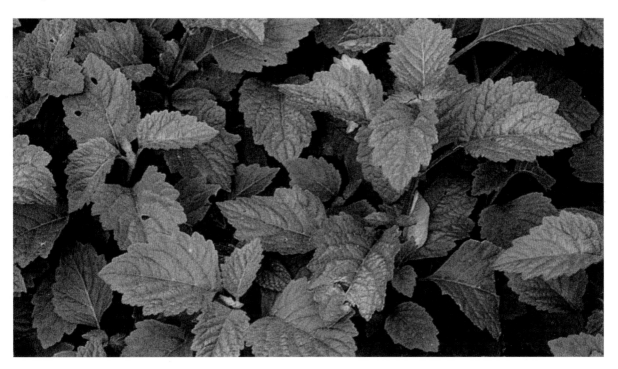

Bergamot
Citrus bergamia

> Bergamot is useful in meditations where depression is deep, wintry, gloomy, and enervating. Though sedative and calming, it has the ability to lift the spirits, and relieves fatigue and exhaustion.

THE CITY OF BERGAMO IN Lombardy, Italy, lends its name to this citrus fruit, which is thought to be a hybrid of bitter orange and lemon. It should not be confused with the herb of the same name. It has never been successfully grown anywhere else in the world, but has been used in Italian folk medicine regularly, mostly for cases of fever. It is boldly yang and consequently is ruled by the sun.

Bergamot is most effective in dealing with depression, anxiety, nervous tension, emotional imbalance, and fear. "In helping with mental and psychological states, Bergamot is almost the most valuable oil... It is often described as uplifting and I cannot improve on this description" (Patricia Davis: *Aromatherapy: An A–Z*).

In cold, gray winter many of us experience a mild form of Seasonal Affective Disorder (SAD), and a few unfortunate people are affected badly and become clinically depressed. Bergamot is of great value in such cases, and perhaps the essential oil derived from the fruit "remembers" the sun that ripened it and is able to express some of this quality.

Bergamot is useful in meditations where depression is deep, wintry, gloomy, and enervating. Though sedative and calming, it has the ability to lift the spirits, and relieves fatigue and exhaustion. Bergamot has a sunny disposition that helps people regain self-confidence; the fragrance is heart-warming and evokes joy. Bergamot would make an ideal ritual offering at the spring equinox, heralding the return of the sun.

However, we must be careful of using bergamot in sunlight. It is a photosensitizer; in other words it increases the skin's reaction to sunlight, so should never be worn on skin that will be exposed to direct sunlight. It is much better to use its sunny qualities without the sun!

Bergamot, the finest of the citrus oils, is used to flavor Earl Grey tea, is a major ingredient of Eau de Cologne, and is used in many other perfumes. It has sweet, lemon fresh top notes and warm, sunny, almost floral, balsamic undertones; it blends beautifully with most oils.

Lemon

Citrus limon

> Lemon essential oil is depurative and detoxifying—helping cleanse the blood and the rest of the body—and it is no surprise that it replicates this effect on the mind.

LEMONS HAVE SOME QUITE unfortunate associations that reflect its sour reputation. In a popular song, the tree and the flower are sweet, but not so the fruit. However, it is generally regarded as something of a cure-all and all-in-one beauty aid in many folk herbal traditions, yet its psychological benefits often seem to have been overlooked. Lemon is most helpful in preventing emotional outbursts.

Lemon trees grow freely in many Mediterranean countries, but the finest lemon oil comes from Sicily. Lemon is yang and ruled by Mercury. Lemon essential oil is depurative and detoxifying–helping cleanse the blood and the rest of the body–and it is no surprise that it replicates this effect on the mind. Tests in Japan found that lemon oil helps concentration by clearing the mind and helping the decision-making process.

This oil is indicated in meditations when the mind is foggy and confused, and clarity is sought; lemon helps shed light on dubious situations and during times of psychological trauma. It is useful in rituals for purification and psychic cleansing. Despite the horrible synthetic lemon aroma found in various cleaning products, the scent of pure lemon is unmistakable: clean, fresh, light, and citrus. Lemon can help rescue a blend of oils that has gone wrong, and mixes easily with other oils.

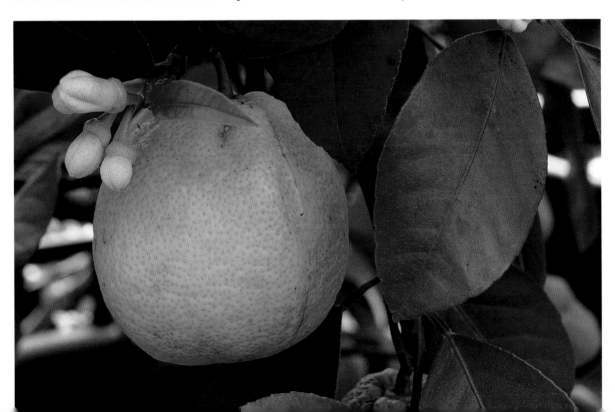

Neroli/Orange Blossom
Citrus bigaradia

ORANGE BLOSSOM OIL WAS introduced to Italian society by Anna Maria de la Tremoille, Princess of Nerole, in the seventeenth century. She loved the fragrance and used it extensively; it soon became fashionable and was called neroli in her honor. Despite having marked feminine qualities, neroli is yang and ruled by the sun.

Neroli is the Rescue Remedy of essential oils and is unsurpassed for dealing with shock, hysteria, and nervous tension. It has a powerful psychological effect, reaching deep into the psyche to bring calm and stability. It is also an aphrodisiac, and this combination of properties led to its traditional inclusion in wedding bouquets, because the fragrance would calm the bride and allow her to enjoy her wedding night.

An excellent sedative and antidepressant, neroli calms and slows the mind, allowing thoughts to clear and settle. For those who are oversensitive, neroli can strengthen their inner being and act like a psychic shield. It has a tonic effect on the heart and is indicated when fear arises with no known cause, and for those who become agitated without good reason. The corresponding physical symptom of diarrhea brought on by shock or fear is also alleviated by neroli.

After an exhausting and emotionally taxing day, a ritual bath with neroli is of great benefit—bringing tranquillity and promoting restful sleep. Before a test or exam, a meditation with neroli will strengthen the

> An excellent sedative and antidepressant, neroli calms and slows the mind, allowing thoughts to clear and settle.

nerves and reduce anxiety, by calming racing thoughts, deepening shallow breathing, and slowing a quickened heartbeat. After the meditation, an affirmation and ritual anointing with neroli will help you face whatever lies ahead.

Neroli is gentle but powerful, and sometimes smells better diluted than straight from the bottle, when it can seem too intense. The delightful fragrance has fresh, light, floral top notes and warm, heady, sweet undertones, and it enriches blends.

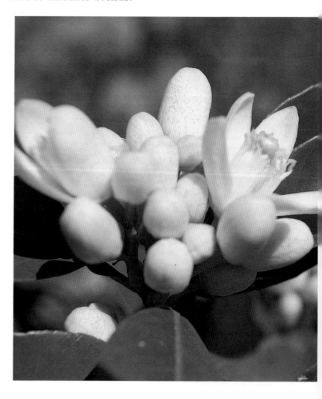

Geranium

Pelargonium gravolens

Geranium is indicated when we need to find harmony and balance in our lives. It is useful in rituals to do with life changes.

GERANIUM IS A GREAT balancer and is indicated when you feel unbalanced, indecisive, or rigid. It is a stimulant of the adrenal cortex, which secretes hormones that govern the balance of other hormones in the body. Geranium naturally balances fluctuating hormone levels and is most helpful for PMS and menopausal symptoms. As an antidepressant sedative it simultaneously balances the accompanying emotional mood swings, calming irritation, and promoting harmony. Some aromatherapists suggest that it should not be used during pregnancy.

Geranium is described as yin and being ruled by Venus, but is almost neutral and has a slight yang warming quality. This makes geranium useful when our inner yin and yang aspects need harmonizing and centering; it allows women to express their masculinity and men their femininity. It helps us to retreat when we are too open, and to be expansive when we are too inward-looking.

Rovesti used geranium successfully in clinically treating anxiety, and it has an uplifting quality similar to bergamot. Geranium is indicated when we need to find harmony and balance in our lives. It is useful in rituals to do with life changes, such as the onset of menstruation or menopause, and helps these transitions flow smoothly.

Geranium has fresh, light, green top notes and soft, floral undertones. It smells a little like rose and is used in the perfume industry to make rose go farther. Its neutral chameleonlike qualities enable geranium to blend with almost any other oil.

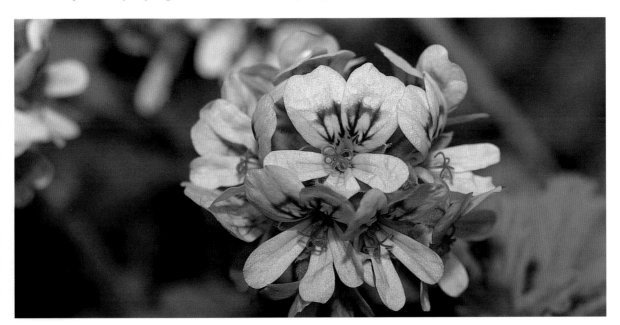

Mandarin

Citrus reticulata

> Other than its uplifting, warming, cheering effects, mandarin's main use in meditations and rituals is for its slightly hypnotic action.

MANDARINS MAY HAVE originated in China—the name comes from the traditional offering of the fruit to the mandarins, the ancient rulers of China. The mandarin tree is now cultivated throughout the Mediterranean and the United States, although it is usually called tangerine in the United States. Consequently, the two essential oils are sometimes confused, though they smell quite different, but mandarin is generally considered to have finer qualities.

The effects of mandarin are similar to those of both neroli and orange, and, in common with all citrus essential oils, the main quality of mandarin is its cheering, uplifting action. It is excellent when combined with neroli, because the synergy seems to be even more effective than either oil on its own. Both oils are very safe, so this is a good blend to use if you are pregnant.

Other than its uplifting, warming, cheering effects, mandarin's main use in meditations and rituals is for its slightly hypnotic action. This makes it the first choice when your mind is overactive, or there is difficulty in switching off and letting go of the day's events. Mandarin gently soothes the mind and promotes a good night's sleep.

These uplifting and hypnotic effects also make mandarin useful in the daytime, particularly in meditations and rituals where you need to clear your mind of old thoughts and issues, literally to blow away the cobwebs.

Mandarin is also a tonic and has a strengthening effect, so is helpful with depression when this is associated with weakness, fragility, and lack of inspiration. Mandarin appeals to our youthful side and is fresh and uplifting.

Mandarin has a sweet citrus aroma, with refreshing, clean top notes and almost floral, surprisingly deep undertones. It is excellent in blends, bringing a refreshing note, but with subtle hidden depths.

Sweet Orange

Citrus sinensis

"I recall a little grove of orange trees, At the gates of Bliddah, it is there that they were beautiful! In the dark, shiny, glossy foliage, The fruits were brilliant as colored glass And gilded the air about with that halo of splendor Which surrounds the radiant flowers."

ALPHONSE DAUDET

ORANGES WERE FIRST cultivated in China, and dried orange peel featured in their medical treatments for coughs and colds. Orange groves are now familiar in temperate climates around the world, but the finest orange oil comes from Sicily. Like all citrus essential oils, orange is simply expressed from the peel.

Orange is known as the "smiley oil"—it conveys warmth, joy, and lightheartedness. Together with lavender it is one of the more popular essential oils and favored by beginners and children. Orange shares the uplifting qualities of bergamot.

Orange is useful in meditations when we are taking ourselves too seriously. It allows us to smile and laugh, and to open up to embrace the world.

Orange reduces fear of the unknown and is indicated in rituals for life's transitions, helping us let go of old obsessions and to move on in life.

When we are emotionally confused, orange helps us to find harmony and to see the bright side of life. It also awakens creativity and is good in rituals that help us to express our creative ideas. The warmth and radiance of orange will cheer you up when life seems dull and gray.

The fragrance of orange is so familiar it needs little description, but a good orange oil has sweet, fresh, fruity top notes with more sensuous, radiant undertones. It blends well with many oils, especially spices, when its uplifting qualities are set alight.

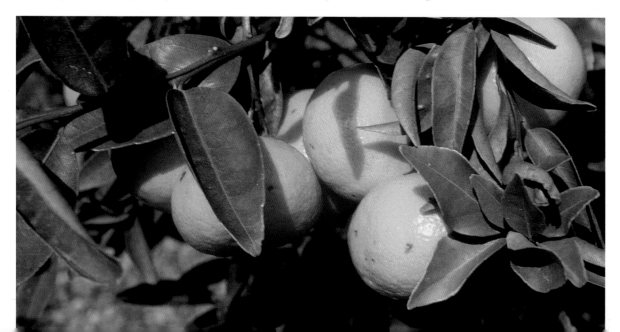

Myrrh

Commiphora myrrha

> Traditionally myrrh was used as an offering to the gods, and was a gift to Jesus, as well as a major ingredient in *megaleion*—a renowned Greek fragrance—and other perfumes.

THE ARABIC WORD *MURR*, meaning bitter, is the origin of the name *myrrh*, though Greek legend states that myrrh emanated from the tears of Myrrha when her father, King Cinyrus of Cyprus, was turned into a shrub.

Myrrh is one of the oldest plant aromatics and was in popular use in the ancient civilizations of Greece and Egypt, as well as in ancient China. A strongly yang oil, myrrh is sometimes ascribed the sun as its ruling planet. However, if we look at the properties of myrrh alongside the legend of Myrrha's tears, there is another strong planetary indication. Myrrh's yang qualities of opening and drying—used to heal wounds—are balanced by its yin anti-inflammatory action. Together with Myrrha's bitter tears of grief, and myrrh's sense of antiquity—literally "old father time"—these qualities all indicate the influence of Saturn.

This makes myrrh invaluable for meditations and rituals where there is bitterness, coming to terms with a lesson hard learned, or working with issues over a long time.

The essential oil is distilled from a gum that oozes from cuts in the bark of a gnarled bush in the desert. The myrrh bush is very hardy—it thrives in the desert, reflecting how myrrh essential oil is tough, but supportive when life seems hard to take.

Traditionally myrrh was used as an offering to the gods, and was a gift to Jesus, as well as a major ingredient in *megaleion*—a renowned Greek fragrance—and other perfumes. In addition, myrrh was carried by soldiers going into battle, as an ancient Greek first-aid kit; soldiers would apply it to their wounds.

Myrrh has musky, smoky top notes with bitter, balsamic incense undertones. On its own it can smell bitter and pungent, but when blended with sweeter, lighter oils it gives a wonderful grounding note. Myrrh should be avoided during pregnancy.

Benzoin

Styrax benzoin

> Benzoin is indicated in meditations where there is sadness and loneliness, particularly where these are chronic or recurrent. It is invaluable in rituals for grief and bereavement.

WHEREAS ORANGE IS KNOWN as the "smiley oil," benzoin is known as the "cuddly oil," and has a comforting, warming effect. The oil is distilled from a gum that comes from trees grown in Thailand and Vietnam (Benzoin Siam) and from Sumatra (Benzoin Sumatra). Like frankincense and myrrh, benzoin is a traditional ingredient of incense, and the smoke of burning it was traditionally used to drive away evil spirits.

Twentieth-century Austrian aromatherapy pioneer Marguerite Maury described benzoin as creating a kind of euphoria, and interposing a padded zone between ourselves and what happens around us. In this way benzoin comforts those who are fragile and alienated, and, combined with its ability to drive away evil spirits, it has a surprising power underneath its sweet surface. Benzoin is yang and ruled by the sun.

Benzoin is indicated in meditations where there is sadness and loneliness, particularly when these are chronic or recurrent. It is invaluable in rituals for grief and bereavement, whether related to a death or the loss of a relationship or career. Benzoin is also useful when dealing with anxiety and depression.

Benzoin is a great comforter and acts like a shield against outside events and disturbances. It is good in rituals and meditations to help let go of old resentments and griefs, and it promotes acceptance and contentment. The symbol of benzoin as a shield also makes it useful in protection rituals, and for psychic detoxification. In aromatherapy, benzoin is used in skin care, especially for chapped hands and mature skin, and the symbol for benzoin (a shield) also applies to protecting the skin.

Benzoin may be a familiar smell from childhood; it is the main ingredient of Friar's Balsam used in inhalations for colds. Benzoin has vanilla ice cream top notes with molasses, balsamic undertones. It is a good fixative and blends well.

> "On the psychological plane, as with many essential oils, we find a parallel with its physical properties—warming, soothing, and stimulating. I use Benzoin to help people who are sad and lonely, depressed or anxious… We might perhaps see here an echo of its former use to 'cast out devils,' for what are the devils of our time, if not such psychological states as these?"
> **PATRICIA DAVIS: *AROMATHERAPY: AN A–Z***

Jasmine
Jasminum officinale

> Although it is a sedative, jasmine's powerful yang nature makes it warming and strengthening; it is certainly not an oil for inaction!

JASMINE IS THE UNDISPUTED king of essential oils. Unfortunately it is also one of the most expensive; it takes about 3.5 million flowers to yield one pound (0.45 kg) of essential oil. Jasmine flowers undergo a chemical change at sunset and the odor intensifies after dark, so the flowers must be picked at this time. It is yang and ruled by Jupiter and is associated with intuitive wisdom.

Jasmine works powerfully on our emotions and is one of the few oils that can produce a euphoric effect. This is not only enjoyable but also increases confidence, inspiration, and optimism. Jasmine is an aphrodisiac, and useful not only for heightening sexual response but also in helping frigidity and impotence. It is both sedative and antidepressant, so it can also relieve the underlying tensions that cause sexual difficulties.

Although it is a sedative, jasmine's powerful yang nature makes it warming and strengthening; it is certainly not an oil for inaction! Jasmine is therefore useful in intimate massage between lovers when there are feelings of insecurity or inadequacy. Jasmine promotes wild abandon and helps you find natural sexual instincts that may have been "civilized" away. It is the best choice for use in rituals to inspire confidence and strength, especially when you feel weak rather than just in need of a boost.

Jasmine is indicated in meditations when there is an unresolved emotional block, when you feel cold and detached, listless, or fearful. Jasmine acts as a tonic on the nerves and because it is both antidepressant and penetrating, it helps to reach the core of the problem. After meditating, ritual anointing with jasmine surrounds the senses with the delicious fragrance, helping you to move forward and get on with life. Jasmine's sense of mystery helps you to allow life to happen freely, without trying to control events.

Smelling jasmine straight from the bottle is not for the fainthearted, but once it is diluted or blended the more subtle notes come through. Jasmine has sweet, floral, exotic top notes with heady, powerful, honey undertones. The fragrance almost seems alive—an indication to treat jasmine with respect. It blends well with light, fresh oils and grounding, earthy oils. Avoid during pregnancy.

Linden/Lime Blossom

Tilia vulgaris

> Linden blossom promotes a deep relaxation and is indicated in meditations for tiredness when stress and an overactive mind are preventing sleep.

LINDEN, OR LIME, BLOSSOMS are a familiar sight in the spring on the grand tree-lined avenues of rural English towns. The flowers are used extensively in herbal medicine, mainly in the form of a tisane or tea, but the essential oil is not yet widely used in aromatherapy. It is to be hoped that now that the essential oil is more readily available, more use will be made of the lovely linden blossom.

Linden blossom—alongside rose, jasmine, neroli, and violet leaf—is an absolute. Absolutes are powerful, highly concentrated, and expensive; a little goes a long way. They are obtained by using a method of solvent extraction, or by using liquid carbon dioxide, when steam distillation would spoil the essential oil.

Linden blossom is good for the nerves and has a calming, sedative, and tonic action. It promotes a deep relaxation and is indicated in meditations for tiredness when stress and an overactive mind prevent sleep. Linden blossom is useful in rituals before stressful activities to calm the nerves, or to deal with hysteria. It can be substituted for neroli, ylang ylang, or jasmine, if the smell is preferred. Linden blossom is also useful after stressful activities, because it soothes the nervous tension accumulated.

The fragrance of linden blossom is calming, and it has sweet, herbaceous, haylike top notes with green, dry, honeyed undertones. It blends easily, especially with citrus and floral oils, and complements the slight bitterness of chamomile and myrrh.

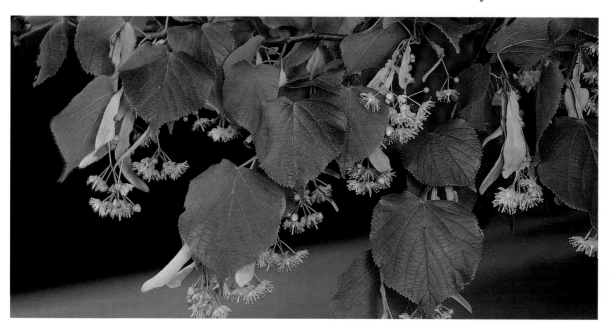

Juniper
Juniperus communis

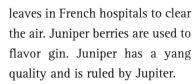

As a traditional ingredient of incense, juniper is useful in all meditations and helps to clear the mind. It is indicated when your mind needs a spring-clean.

THERE ARE TWO ESSENTIAL oils distilled from the juniper tree; the better oil comes from the berries, rather than the mixture of berries and twigs. Juniper is a traditional ingredient of Tibetan incense, and has long been used in herbal folk remedies for its purifying, diuretic, and disinfectant qualities. As recently as the twentieth century, juniper twigs were burned with rosemary leaves in French hospitals to clear the air. Juniper berries are used to flavor gin. Juniper has a yang quality and is ruled by Jupiter.

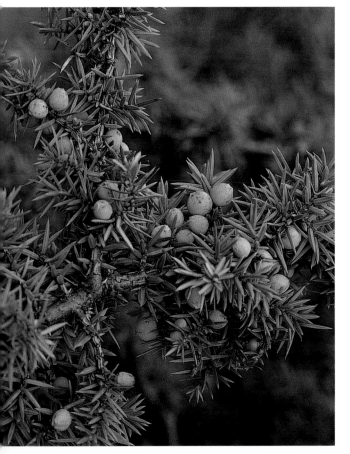

The detoxifying action of juniper on the physical body is well matched with its action psychologically, spiritually, and emotionally. Juniper strengthens and uplifts the spirit when you have low energy, or feel anxious or inadequate. It is the most powerful psychic detoxifying essential oil, and the first choice for psychic cleansing rituals, whether of yourself, or a room or other space. A simple quick ritual for personal psychic cleansing is to rub a couple of drops of juniper between your palms and sweep your hands over your clothed body in swift, long strokes. A longer, but most effective, ritual for personal psychic cleansing is a ritual bath with juniper.

As a traditional ingredient of incense, juniper is useful in all meditations and helps to clear the mind. It is indicated when your mind needs a spring clean, when you feel that contact with other people has disturbed you, or when you seek clarity. If you ritually burn juniper during your first night in a new home, it dispels the psychic presence of the previous occupants.

Juniper has an interesting aroma. You might need to try a few different sources to find one you like because juniper varies more than most essential oils depending on where and when it is grown. It has clean, fresh, turpentine top notes, and smoky, woody undertones. It adds a fresh, clean note to blends. Juniper should be avoided during pregnancy.

Cedarwood

Cedrus atlantica

> Cedarwood was much used in medicine, cosmetics, and perfumery by many older civillizations, alongside its traditional use as incense.

THERE ARE SEVERAL DIFFERENT cedars, but *Cedrus atlantica* is the finest and is closely related to the Cedars of Lebanon mentioned in the Bible. Cedarwood has been used for its aroma since antiquity because the wood contains a high percentage of essential oil. This gives the wood itself many of the properties of the oil, notably its insect repellent powers. Cedarwood was highly prized and honored as a symbol of strength, dignity, and nobility. It is yang and ruled by Uranus.

Cedarwood was much used in medicine, cosmetics, and perfumery by many older civilizations, alongside its traditional use as incense. The ancient Egyptians also used cedarwood for embalming. Cedarwood is held in high esteem, and its symbolic status is easily understood when you realize that cedars grow to over 100 ft (30 m) in height and have been known to live for more than a thousand years.

The properties of the essential oil are mirrored in this majestic tree; there is strength and courage in the fragrance of cedarwood, alongside softness. This makes cedarwood an ideal oil for rituals where courage and dignity are needed. The smell of cedarwood is masculine, and it is much used in men's toiletries. This yang male quality is a useful counterpoint to balance excess yin.

Cedarwood wraps you in its strong, kind arms and helps you find comfort and calm. It is useful in meditations to help reduce fear, and the aggression born from fear. It is an appropriate essential oil to burn as an offering to the gods, and the Temple of Solomon was built from finest cedar.

Cedarwood has warm, soft, camphorlike top notes and sweet, rich, balsamic undertones.

It should be blended with discretion, but is useful in traditionally masculine blends. Cedarwood should be avoided during pregnancy.

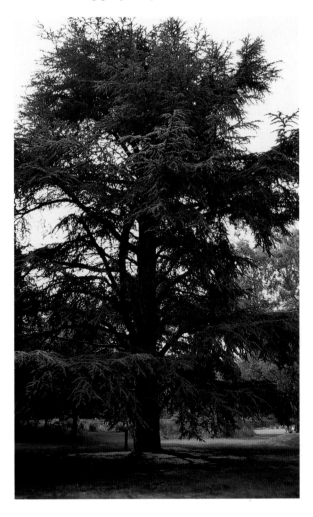

Melissa
Melissa officinalis

> *"[Melissa] causeth the mind and heart to become merry, and reviveth the heart, faintings and swoonings, especially of such who are overtaken in sleep, and driveth away all troublesome cares and thoughts out of the mind arising from melancholy"*
>
> **NICHOLAS CULPEPER: CULPEPER'S COMPLETE HERBAL**

ALSO KNOWN AS LEMON BALM, or balm, the word *melissa* originates from the Greek for bee, because bees are particularly attracted to the nectar for making honey. Paracelsus, the sixteenth-century German physician, called melissa the elixir of life, and the Arab Persian physician Avicenna (980–1037CE) described it as strengthening the spirit, making a happy heart, and chasing away dark thoughts. Melissa is yang and ruled by Jupiter.

Although the herb grows prolifically, melissa is expensive because of its high water and low essential oil content. Beware of cheap melissa; it will be lemongrass or citronella and lack the properties of true melissa. Despite the cost, melissa is one of the most useful oils for shock, depression, grief, and anxiety; it enhances life.

Melissa is valuable in meditations when we have lost our center or perhaps our inner direction. It has a tonic effect on the heart, strengthening the heart chakra, and is indicated for use in meditations after sudden shock. Melissa helps us find inner contentment by calming a troubled mind and gladdening the spirit.

Melissa is a powerful ally for those suffering from sudden grief, such as losing someone close in an accident. It is indicated in a ritual to lessen the shock and allow natural grieving to flow. Eventually it helps us to come to terms with our loss, and to rediscover the light in life when we are ready.

When melancholy and lethargy arise for no reason, using melissa in an anointing perfume will surround us with its joyous fragrance and help lift our spirits. Melissa can be used to help anxiety and nervous tension instead of neroli if the fragrance is preferred. In aromatherapy, melissa is used to help both asthma and eczema, where it works by reducing the stress that contributes to these conditions.

Melissa has warm, fresh, lemon sherbet top notes and sweet, radiant, delicate, balsamic, herbal undertones. It is the most subtle of the lemon-scented essential oils and blends easily.

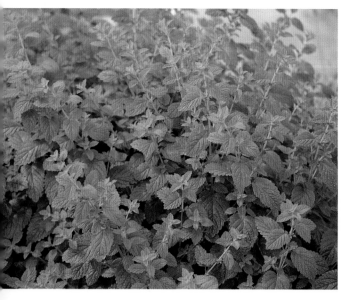

Angelica

Angelica archangelica

YOU MAY BE FAMILIAR WITH candied angelica, the green decorations on cakes and pastries, but angelica essential oil is far more interesting. In the Middle Ages, angelica was used to prevent infections, and Paracelsus cited its use against bubonic plague. As well as being strongly antiviral, angelica has pronounced yang qualities and works by strengthening the mind and spirit; it doesn't let you give up.

Angelica is indicated for use in rituals to increase perseverance when there is a sense of hopelessness or indecision. By helping us reconnect with our soul—our guardian angel—angelica helps us find our inner power to move forward. Angelica was used in many alchemical formulas for extending life, or increasing life force, and is useful for longevity rituals. Angelica

> When we feel afraid and timid, angelica is indicated for use in meditations to balance and soothe weakness and faintheartedness. It helps us to regenerate body and spirit.

helps us to increase our awareness of the angelic realms and to be receptive to divine forces. Angelica is useful in intimate massage blends for lovers, because it fortifies sexual desire; it is also indicated for helping frigidity.

When we feel afraid and timid, angelica is indicated for use in meditations to balance and soothe weakness and faintheartedness. It helps us to regenerate body and spirit by healing, calming, and balancing our nervous system. Its use in convalescence indicates its powers to help when recovering from emotional pain or spiritual crisis.

Angelica has spicy, rich top notes with fresh, earthy, herbaceous undertones. It is an ingredient of Chartreuse and Benedictine liqueurs. It must be blended with care; too much can be overpowering.

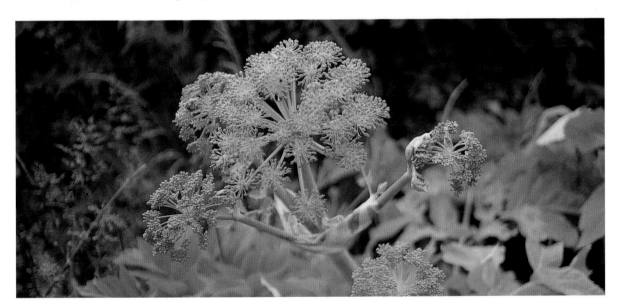

Basil/Holy Basil

Ocimum basilicum/sanctum

BASIL IS KNOWN AS THE ROYAL herb, from the Greek *basilikos* meaning royal. It is called *tulsi* in India, and is dedicated to the god Vishnu, and regarded as the incarnation of his wife, Lakshmi, the goddess of fortune and beauty. Basil is used widely in Ayurvedic medicine and religious rituals. Corpses are washed with basil-infused water, and a basil leaf is placed on the chest of the dead. Tulsi leaves are hung over the front doorway of houses belonging to followers of Vishnu to protect from evil spirits. Basil is yang and ruled by Mars.

> *"I adore tulsi, whose roots are the journey's end of any pilgrimage, whose stem is the abode of the gods."*
>
> **OLD INDIAN PRAYER**

One of the predominant properties of basil is its ability to strengthen the mind, aid concentration, and give clarity. This complements its tonic effect on the nervous system, making it an excellent choice to deal with mental fatigue and indecision, especially when these are chronic and have caused weakness.

Basil works sensitively in rituals for psychic protection, when subtlety is required. This mirrors its traditional medical use as a prophylactic in India against colds and flu. Basil is not as powerful an antiseptic as thyme or rosemary, and has a more subtle effect, which is useful in long-term treatment. This points toward using basil when psychic protection is needed over a long period of time.

Basil is indicated for use in meditations to stimulate mental activity and to clear the mind. The African Soussou name for basil is *barikiri*—meaning devil chaser—and if we regard negative, repetitive thoughts as devils, we can see how basil helps chase these away. It is the least sharp of the cephalic (mental stimulant) oils, and its gentle antidepressive, tonic action makes it pleasant to use.

Basil has sweet, green, herbaceous top notes and spicy, licorice undertones. Holy basil has more depth. Both blend surprisingly easily, particularly with lavender, frankincense, narcissus, and lemon. Avoid during pregnancy.

Rosemary

Rosmarinus officinalis

ROSEMARY HAS BEEN USED AS an incense and to drive out evil spirits since antiquity; one of its names is *incensier*. As we learn from Ophelia (*see* right), rosemary is for remembrance, and it is one of the strongest cephalic (mental stimulant), essential oils. The name comes from the Latin *ros marinus*, meaning sea dew.

Greek and Roman students wore wreaths of rosemary around their brows to help them study, and the fourteenth-century alchemist Raymond Lilly used rosemary oil to attract "good ghosts." Rosemary is a symbol of friendship and love as well as a reminder of life and death; its presence was required at weddings and funerals alike. Rosemary is yang and ruled by the sun.

Rosemary is good for recovering memory loss, and thus useful in regression rituals that seek to uncover early or prebirth experiences. Its pronounced action on the mind makes it useful in meditations to clear the mind of confusion and doubt, especially when there is debility or weakness.

Combined with neroli and applied to the wrists before exams, the calming effect of neroli and the stimulating effect of rosemary strengthen the mind and increase creativity.

It is useful in meditations where there is emotional pain in the heart. If grief causes apathy, rosemary helps to cut through blocked emotions and move on. It helps with physical and psychological headaches. It has sharp, fresh, green top notes and herbaceous, camphoraceous undertones. Used with discretion, it blends well. Rosemary should be avoided during pregnancy.

> " 'There's rosemary; that's for remembrance,' says Ophelia... but the memory that rosemary brings is not only earthly; it also calls on us to remember our celestial home and our divine origins, and the smoke from burning it accompanies our souls to the gates of Heaven."
>
> **PHILIPPE MAILHEBIAU: PORTRAITS IN OILS**

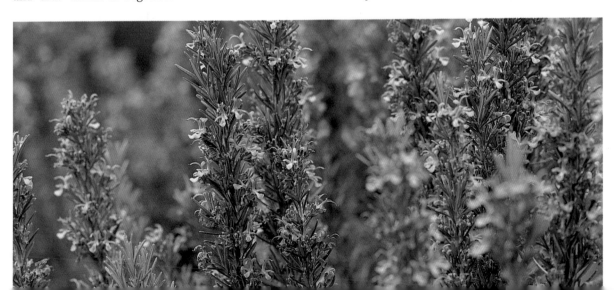

Black Pepper

Piper nigrum

BLACK PEPPER HAS A WARM character, full of mystery and intrigue, reflecting its oriental origins. One of the oldest known spices, Black Pepper's name comes from the Sanskrit *pippali*. A certain order of mendicant monks (i.e. those supported by alms) in India who traveled extensively by foot used to swallow whole seven to nine grains of pepper a day, which reportedly gave them remarkable endurance. Black pepper is a stimulating essential oil, working as much on the emotions and the psyche as on the body and mind. It is very yang and ruled by Mars.

> In meditations to build strength and endurance, black pepper is one of the most valuable essential oils. It fortifies the mind and spirit—the image of stoking a fire springs to mind. After the meditation, anointing with perfume including black pepper will boost you.

In his *Botanicum Officinale*, published in 1722, the herbalist Joseph Miller recommends black pepper for "cold affections of the nerves," because it warms and strengthens psychologically. It is indicated for use in rituals when you feel cold, aloof, and detached. It helps you to reconnect and dispels alienation.

It is best used blended in ritual baths, where the warmth of water, use of candles, and so on reinforce its action.

Black pepper is also useful in intimate massage between lovers who have lost the heat of passion, and it has a slight aphrodisiac quality. However, its action is much more holistic and subtle than just sexually stimulating, and it works by warming the underlying emotions, allowing your feelings to flow.

In meditations to build strength and endurance, black pepper is one of the most valuable essential oils we can use. It fortifies the mind and spirit—the image of stoking a fire springs to mind. After the meditation, a ritual anointing with a perfume including black pepper will boost you with its resolute quality.

Black pepper has hot, spicy, fiery top notes and sharp, woody undertones. As with all the spice oils, use black pepper sparingly and in low dilutions to avoid skin irritation. It blends beautifully and is a good fixative, giving a mysterious Oriental quality to perfumes.

Ginger
Zingiber officinale

> *Ginger's character is described as: "arousing and warm, fortifying and opulent, inviting and satisfying."*
>
> **VALERIE ANN WORWOOD, AROMATHERAPIST**

CHINESE MEDICINE USES ginger extensively for its powerful healing properties. Originally native to Asia, ginger came to Europe via the Spice Route in the Middle Ages and gained popularity swiftly. As a spice, ginger has obvious warming qualities on both mind and body. However, it is principally used when there is excess moisture, and it has a pronounced drying effect, demonstrating its yang properties.

Ginger is indicated in rituals and meditations when there is debility through nervous exhaustion. It warms and strengthens the emotions. In the same way as it can dry excess moisture on the physical plane, ginger helps to dry tears of frustrated exhaustion. Ginger is especially good in cold, damp weather when you feel depressed; its warmth cuts through the winter blues.

A traditional remedy for nausea, ginger can help with butterflies in the stomach, or when nervousness makes you feel sick. Blended with neroli or melissa, ginger empowers you to "feel the fear and do it anyway." Ginger is useful in rituals to build courage to move into action. It can also renew passion for a cause and can be described as a psychic, physical, and sexual energizer.

Ginger has a reputation as an aphrodisiac. Powdered ginger root is woven into belts by Senegalese women to invigorate their men's virility. It is indicated in intimate massage between lovers when there is tiredness or boredom; blended with jasmine, ginger is stimulating and helps you find your wild side.

Aromatherapist Valerie Ann Worwood describes ginger as "arousing and warm, fortifying and opulent, inviting and satisfying," which sums up its character rather well.

Fresh root ginger is used to flavor food and in ginger tea for its excellent digestive properties. It has sharp, green top notes and fiery, woody, sweet, spicy undertones. It is fantastic in blends when used carefully.

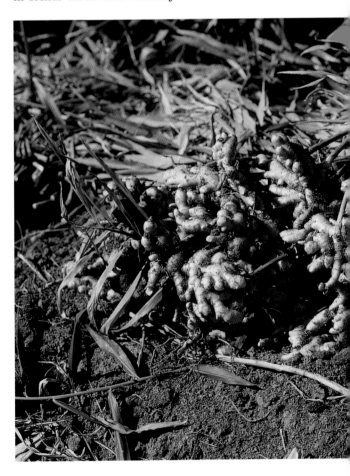

Rose

Rosa centifolia/damascena

ROSE IS THE QUEEN OF essential oils as jasmine is the king. It is one of the oldest and most precious essential oils, as well as the most symbolic. Legends abound, but essentially the rose symbolizes life, death, and the resurrection; the wounds of Christ, the transmutation of his blood, and the Holy Grail that collected it. Roses are associated with Venus and Aphrodite; it is said the rose was originally white, only becoming pink when Venus pricked her foot on a thorn. Rose is yin and ruled by Venus.

> *"Roses put to the nose to smell do comfort the brain and the heart and quickeneth the spirit."*
>
> **BANCKE'S HERBAL**

The value of rose cannot be overestimated, and if you can afford only one of the expensive oils, this is the one. Roses are symbols of love and valuable in all love's aspects. When wounded in love, anointing with rose will assist healing; it is a tonic for the heart physically as well as emotionally. In the first flush of love, rose will honor and celebrate your union.

Rose strengthens the sexual organs; it is an aphrodisiac, a cleansing tonic for the uterus, and it increases semen. This gives rose pride of place in intimate massage between lovers when there is frigidity or impotence, especially when these arise from fear, or past feelings of being hurt. Rose also has deep psychological properties; it balances, comforts, and opens doors to love and sexuality.

Rose is invaluable in rituals concerned with death and dying; it reduces fear and brings out wisdom, easing the transition between life and death. For the bereaved, rose soothes and helps people to come to terms with loss, and it is beneficial in meditations on death. Rose is a powerful antidepressant and is useful in meditations and rituals to help lift the spirits while acknowledging and soothing pain, sadness, and depression.

The different roses share a similar scent. Rose is simply divine, with sweet, floral top notes and deep, honeyed undertones. Even one drop will transform a blend into something special. Avoid during the first three months of pregnancy.

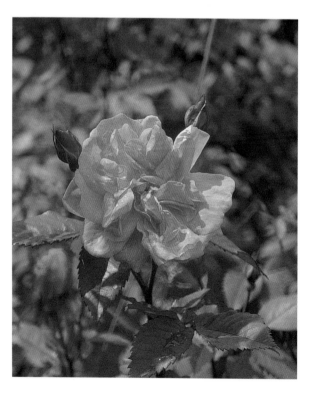

Narcissus

Narcissus poeticus

> Narcissus is soporific, causing you to feel languid and relaxed. If you are overexcited, or hysterical, its sedative, hypnotic, earthy quality is deeply calming.

NARCISSUS WAS ONE OF THE essential oils distilled by the Arabs for use in perfumes. The name comes from the Greek *narkao*, which means "to be numb," and narcissus has a pronounced narcotic action, so must be used with great care. Narcissus is used in India as an anointing oil before going into the temple for prayers and meditation.

The legend of the Greek god Narcissus is interesting in terms of the essential oil. As a handsome young god, Narcissus fell in love with his own image, reflected in a pool belonging to the nymph Echo. She caused the water nymphs who lived there to seize his soul, whereupon he died and sprang up as a spring flower.

This reveals the character of narcissus as inward-looking, and this essential oil is indicated for use in meditations and rituals when introspection is required. Narcissus is narcotic and also soporific, causing you to feel languid and relaxed. If you are overexcited, or hysterical, its sedative, hypnotic, earthy quality is deeply calming and grounding.

Narcissus is also gently aphrodisiac and makes an interesting and sensual addition to blends for lovers. Narcissus has heady, herbaceous, green top notes with sweet, floral, mysterious undertones. It enhances blends, reflecting its use in the perfume industry. It should be used very carefully and only in small amounts.

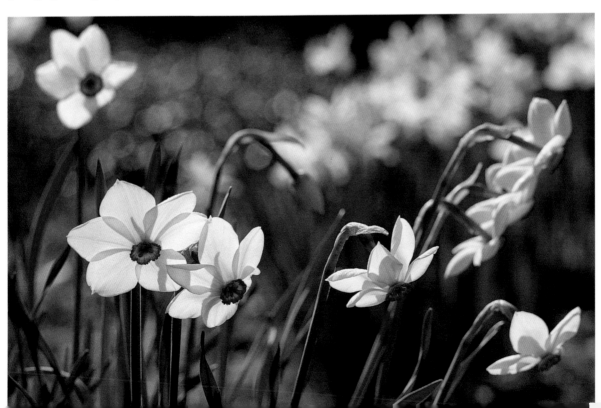

Clary Sage

Salvia sclarea

> "Some brewers of Ale and Beere do put it in their drinke to make it more heady, fit to please drunkards."
>
> **SEVENTEENTH-CENTURY WRITER**

THE NAME OF THIS HERB comes from "clear-eye," because a traditional mucilage made from the seeds was used as an eye-wash to reduce inflammation of the eye. Other traditional uses include the fortification of wine and beer; in Germany it is known as muscatel sage. Clary sage is yang and ruled by the planet Mercury.

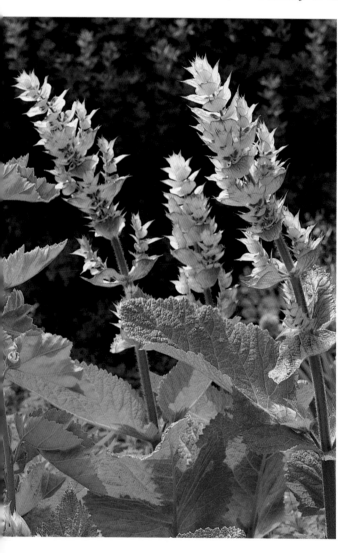

Clary sage is perhaps the most euphoric essential oil, and it has been described as giving a druglike "high." This makes it valuable in rituals when you seek divine inspiration from the spiritual or astral planes. It works by allowing us to temporarily move beyond our usual ego identification and to be receptive to outside influences.

In meditations to lift the spirits, clary sage is also useful, because it is a powerful antidepressant. Less would be used for this purpose than for a ritual, and clary sage would be blended with noneuphoric oils in order to maintain concentration. Clary sage helps in meditations when you feel paranoid, hysterical, or debilitated, because it is a powerful sedative and nerve tonic.

The euphoric effect of clary sage is linked to its aphrodisiac quality, so this is another useful oil for intimate massage, especially when there are inhibitions, or excessive sensitivity. It is helpful with painful periods and menopausal symptoms, and combined with its other qualities, it is therefore appropriate for use in rituals about the onset and cessation of menstruation.

Clary sage has sweet herbaceous top notes and nutty almost floral undertones. It is a good fixative and blends well. Clary sage should be avoided during pregnancy, and it is best to avoid using it shortly before drinking alcohol. Do not drive immediately after using clary sage. Do not confuse clary sage with common sage, which can be toxic.

Sweet Marjoram

Origanum majorana

> The great comforter of the essential oils, marjoram helps with pain on all levels. There is something special about its warming and comforting effect, and it is very good for grief.

MARJORAM IS A TRADITIONAL European herbal remedy, and the ancient Greeks used it in perfumes and medicines. There are various species, and the name *oregano* comes from a Greek word meaning "joy of the mountain." Marjoram is yang and ruled by the planet Mercury.

The great comforter of the essential oils, marjoram helps with pain on all levels. There is something special about the warming and comforting effect of marjoram, and it is very good for grief. Marjoram has a warming, comforting effect on the heart, and calms hysteria. However, its action is slightly numbing—giving you an extra "skin" when you feel too sensitive—so care must be taken not to overuse marjoram to the point where it dulls your senses.

Marjoram is indicated in meditations and rituals to do with bereavement and grief, especially the death of a partner or the end of a relationship. Psychologically, marjoram warms and comforts, and on a physical level it reduces sexual desire, a quality known as anaphrodisiac. This quality makes it useful when you choose to be celibate, and is helpful during meditation retreats.

Though obviously not a sexy oil, marjoram is indicated for use in intimate massage when one partner wishes to nurture and comfort the other, perhaps after a long, tiring, stressful day. Intimate massage with a loved one need not be sexual, and deepens the caring aspect of a relationship. Marjoram is particularly useful in this context, because it works well at relaxing tight, aching muscles. As a consequence of this, marjoram is useful in ritual bathing, perhaps blended with a psychic detoxifying oil.

Marjoram essential oil has spicy, herbaceous top notes and warm, woody undertones. A good marjoram essential oil is subtle, rather than too camphoraceous or sharp, and it tends to blend well in small amounts. It should be avoided during pregnancy.

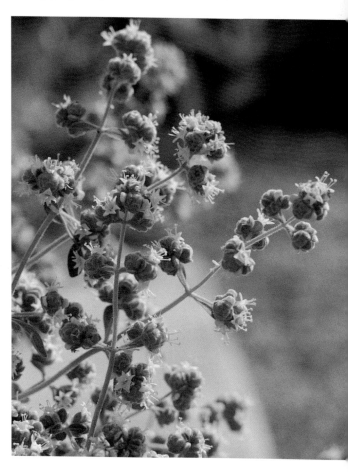

Sandalwood

Santalum album

> Sandalwood is an aphrodisiac, excellent in blends for intimate massage, bringing harmony and joy.

SANDALWOOD HAS THE LONGEST history of religious use in incense of all the aromatics. It is also used extensively in perfumes, cosmetics, and medicine. The best sandalwood comes from Mysore in India, and is superior to the Chinese variety. Indian saddhus, or holy men, wear sandalwood paste on their foreheads as a sign of religious practice. It is ritually burned on funeral pyres, and also at Hindu weddings, where sandalwood fumes from the sacred fire bless the union. Sandalwood is yang and ruled by Uranus.

Chakras are the natural energy centers of the body, connected by subtle channels known as

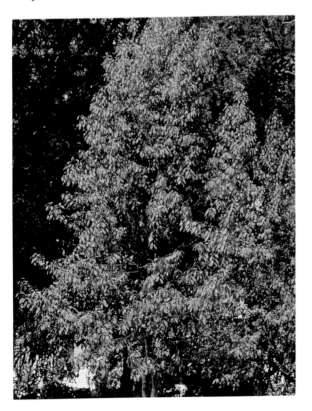

meridians and used in acupuncture. The main chakras are root, navel, solar plexus, heart, throat, brow, and crown. In certain yogic traditions sandalwood is ascribed to both the root chakra (sexuality) and the crown chakra (wisdom and insight). This apparent contradiction is dispelled with the realization that sandalwood is used to arouse kundalini. This is the Indian tantric concept of arousing sexual energy for the purpose of transmutation into spiritual wisdom. It is also considered the perfume of the subtle body or aura (the energy field surrounding living beings).

Sandalwood is therefore most useful in rituals that work with transforming our energies in this way. It helps you to balance your energies when the chakras are uneven; it restores equilibrium. It helps to connect and unite the subtle energy channels and centers, and is truly a sacred fragrance.

The traditional use of sandalwood in incense makes it one of the most appropriate essential oils to burn as an offering to the gods. It is indicated for meditations when your life is too hectic and you need to slow down, particularly when stress is making you irritable or aggressive. Sandalwood's warm, heavy fragrance increases rather than diminishes over time, and it is the most longlasting of the oils.

Sandalwood is an aphrodisiac and consequently is excellent in blends for intimate massage, bringing harmony and joy; it is useful to slow an overquick arousal. Sandalwood has sweet, woody, roselike top notes and balsamic, spicy, oriental undertones. It blends beautifully.

Rosewood
Aniba rosaeodora

> Rosewood is used mainly for spiritual purposes, whether meditation, ritual, or spiritual healing. It has an uplifting, balancing effect and is useful when you are tired.

THERE ARE NO TRADITIONAL therapeutic uses of rosewood essential oil, and the wood was used largely for furniture. In the last few decades rosewood essential oil was in big demand, and deforestation occurred as a result. The tree is now virtually extinct in French Guiana, and numbers have been greatly reduced in Brazil. Efforts by international ecological agencies working with the government in Brazil have produced sustainable rosewood plantations, so ensure your rosewood oil comes from one of these. It is subtly yang and ruled by both the sun and Venus.

Rosewood is used mainly for spiritual purposes, whether meditation, ritual, or spiritual healing. It has an uplifting, balancing effect and is useful when you are tired, especially if there is also nervousness or lack of connection with your inner spirit, or soul. A simple breathing meditation using rosewood and angelica will help you reconnect with the Divine.

Rosewood clears the mind but is not a major stimulant, so it is also calming and steadies the nerves. This makes it useful for rituals at night because it will keep you alert without preventing sleep afterward. In an anointing perfume, rosewood will give endurance. It is has aphrodisiac qualities and, blended with rose, makes an exquisite massage oil for lovers.

Rosewood has a most delicate fragrance, both subtle and powerful. It has soft, floral top notes and sweet, woody undertones. It is very good in blends, especially with other woods, florals, and citrus oils, adding a harmonizing note.

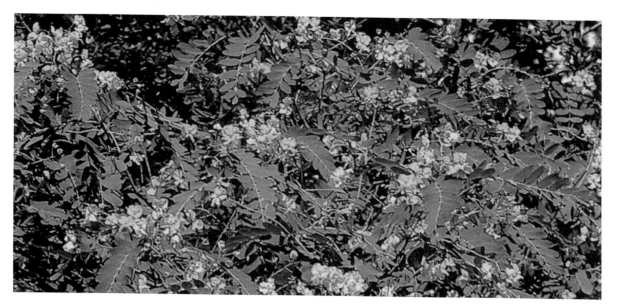

Additional Essential Oils

A KEY FACTOR FOR USING ESSENTIAL OILS IN A sacred context is that you should trust your intuition and inner feelings. Logic and authority may dictate particular oils for a specific meditation or ritual, but they might smell wrong to you. In which case, you must choose your own selection, based on intuition and smell to honor your individuality and the unique occasion of the ceremony.

The essential oils described on the previous pages are a selection that most readily lend themselves for use in meditation and rituals, but there are many others. There is no point using an oil or blend that is recommended if it does not resonate with your soul, so a brief description of some other easily available essential oils follows to expand your options. There are still more not mentioned here, and you can try smelling these in a store that sells essential oils. If anything appeals, buy it and try it!

Elemi (*Canarium luzonicum*)

Elemi was used for embalming by the ancient Egyptians. A close relative of frankincense and myrrh, elemi is a powerful meditation aid that helps you find your center, especially when you need strength and balance. Elemi can be blended with frankincense or myrrh, or used as a substitute if the smell is preferred. It has light, fresh, lemon top notes and spicy, green, balsamic undertones, and it blends easily.

Petitgrain (*Citrus aurantium*)

Petitgrain has many of the same qualities as neroli, yet is much cheaper. Indeed, petitgrain and neroli are distilled from the leaves and twigs of the same tree. A traditional ingredient of cologne, petitgrain is particularly useful for fatigue, because it refreshes mind and spirit. It stimulates the mind, brings joy to

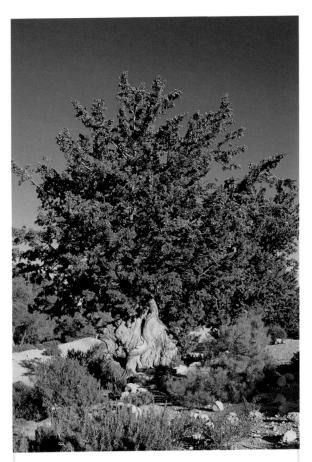

Cypress

Cypress is associated with cemeteries, and both the ancient Egyptians and Romans dedicated the cypress tree to gods of death and the underworld.

the heart, and is generally relaxing and balancing. Petitgrain has fresh, floral, citrus top notes and light, woody undertones. Petitgrain blends easily and can lift a heavy blend.

Cypress (*Cupressus sempevirens*)

Highly prized in both medicine and incense by many ancient civilizations, cypress is still used as a purification incense by the Tibetans. Like juniper, cypress is useful in psychic detoxification rituals and can be blended with juniper or used as a substitute.

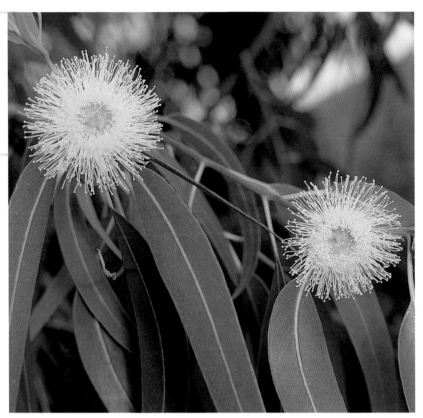

Eucalyptus globulus

Eucalyptus is an effective insect repellant and groves of eucalyptus are planted near swamps in Africa to help prevent the spread of malaria.

It is a powerful astringent and dries up excess fluid; psychologically, it helps dry up excessive speech and thoughts, so is useful in meditations when the mind is overactive. Cypress has spicy, resinous top notes and smoky, balsamic undertones; blend with care. Avoid using during pregnancy.

Palmarosa (*Cymbopogon martinii*)

Palmarosa essential oil is distilled from a grass related to lemongrass. Known as "Nature's copycat," palmarosa is similar to—and is used to "extend"—rose and geranium in the perfume industry, though its aroma clearly lacks the power and depth of rose. Nonetheless, palmarosa is valuable in meditations when stress leaves you feeling vulnerable; it is very gentle and may be preferred to the more powerful oils. Palmarosa has sweet, light, rosy floral top notes and geranium undertones, and it blends well.

Eucalyptus and lemon eucalyptus (*Eucalyptus globulus/citriodora*)

Eucalyptus is an effective insect repellant and groves of eucalyptus are planted near swamps in Africa to help prevent malaria.

Eucalyptus oils have a piercing, fresh, and stimulating effect, demonstrated by their use in inhalations to clear blocked sinuses and stuffy heads. Either type of eucalyptus could be useful in a meditation blend when you have a cold, or feel lethargic; they both help to clear the mind.

Included in a ritual bath in the morning, lemon eucalyptus dispels fatigue and debility and helps you to face the day ahead. Eucalyptus has fresh, sharp, camphoraceous top notes and penetrating undertones. The lemon variety has fresh, citronella lemon top notes and sweet, balsamic undertones. Blend sparingly, unless you like the pungent smell.

Blending

"Creative blending is an aesthetic alchemical process... A blend is not made at once, rather it evolves, it organically grows and interacts not only with the essential oils, but also with the blender."

JOHN STEELE: *INTERNATIONAL JOURNAL OF AROMATHERAPY, VOL II, NO. 2*

ALTHOUGH IT IS SOMETIMES APPROPRIATE TO use one essential oil in a meditation or ritual, often a blend is best. The extensive range of essential oils and the use of different proportions mean that each blend has a unique quality. This reflects the special nature of each blend, and though you may wish to recreate exactly the same blend again, there will always be subtle differences.

A blend is not just a collection of essential oils mixed together. When you make a blend you create more than the sum of the parts. This is called synergy, and reflects how the oils interact with each other, and with yourself. The act of blending is in itself a ceremony, and is the first stage of whatever meditation or ritual you are about to undertake.

Blending is an art and, in common with the other arts, is an intuitive, creative process that finds its highest expression in the art of perfumery. Perfumers use other odiferous material as well as essential oils and work with thousands of individual aromatics. However, even just using essential oils gives us a large range of aromas to choose from, so we need some guidance in the art of blending.

A fragrant harmony

Blending borrows the concept of scales from music, and an ideal blend will have top, middle, and base notes. As we learned with the descriptions of the

Selected blends demonstrating the scale of notes

Blend	top note	middle note	base note
1	lavender	marjoram	benzoin
2	bergamot	jasmine	sandalwood
3	basil	neroli	black pepper
4	chamomile	geranium	cypress
5	rose *(centifolia)*	melissa	frankincense
6	eucalyptus citriodora	clary sage	patchouli
7	mandarin	geranium	patchouli
8	lavender	rose *(damascena)*	frankincense
9	bergamot	ylang ylang	black pepper
10	basil	juniper	frankincense

essential oils, each one is also composed of different notes. These evaporate at different rates, so we smell the different parts at different times. So when we smell a single oil, at first our nose registers one set of aromatic particles, and later others come through; with a blend this becomes more complex and the fragrance subtly changes over time.

Perfumers and aromatherapists learn the various "rules" of blending, but for the purpose of spiritual blends, the best rule is to experiment; whether it works for you is what is important. However, at first limit yourself to three essential oils, and—if you like—have an idea of a light top note, a middle, and a deep base note. Choose your oils from the descriptions, from your own intuition, and from the individual smell.

Before mixing the oils into massage oil or your burner, put a drop of each onto a cotton ball. Then wave them, holding them closely together a little way from your nose; don't sniff too deeply. This allows the oils to diffuse and gives you a good idea of what the blend will smell like. Smell your selection immediately, and also leave it for a few minutes and smell it again. Be aware of what has changed, and remember that your meditation or ritual takes place over time, and that the blend will change subtly over this period.

If it smells awful, try again! If it smells almost right, you will probably sense that one of the three oils needs to be stronger or weaker; this can be changed by using more or fewer drops in the blend. Perhaps one oil needs to be replaced. When your selection feels and smells right, you are ready to create the blend. Let the ceremony begin...

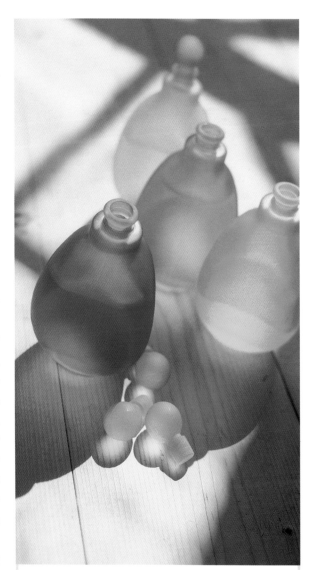

Blending

Blending is an ancient art that seeks to create a harmonious perfume. Having a top, middle, and base note creates a rounded fragrance, although blends for spiritual purposes are personally selected according to intuition.

Creating an Altar with Essential Oils

"In the presence of God people hope to nourish their soul.
This is why priests and priestesses have used fragrances during solemn religious rites and rituals throughout history."

SUZANNE FISCHER-RIZZI:
COMPLETE AROMATHERAPY HANDBOOK

YOU ARE GOING TO USE ESSENTIAL OILS FOR spiritual purposes, so it is a good idea to create an altar. This provides a dedicated sacred place for burning essential oils during meditation and for ritual offerings to the gods. Your altar and the symbols on it act as a conduit between the mundane and spiritual planes.

Placing new bottles of essential oils on your altar for a few days (provided it is not in direct sunlight) before storing them will help attune them to their eventual spiritual use. Once a blend of oils is mixed you can place it on the altar as an offering to enhance the effectiveness by allowing it to absorb the sacred atmosphere.

You can make your altar on a shelf or a low table in a quiet corner of a private room. This helps create a suitable atmosphere for meditation, and will help make a sacred space for ritual. Over time a place used for spiritual work develops its own special energy; we can feel this when we walk into churches and temples.

Placing offerings on your altar

Everything placed on your altar becomes an offering to the gods. If you follow a spiritual tradition you can make your offerings specific to God, Isis, Buddha, or another central figure. Otherwise your offerings can be to Nature's gods and goddesses, or to whatever or whomever you regard as a source of spiritual wisdom.

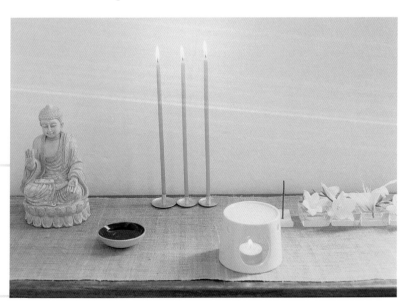

Altar

A simple altar, like the one pictured here, creates a sacred space for your meditations and rituals with essential oils. A few beautiful objects are more precious than too many.

It is the quality of the offerings that is important rather than the quantity, so you don't want to crowd your altar with objects. Like music, the spaces (intervals) are as important as the objects (notes) to create the overall effect, so offering a few beautiful, simple things is appropriate.

Traditional offerings include candles, a small bowl of water, incense, and a few flowers in a vase. As you are going to offer essential oils, these can replace the incense, because they will fulfill the same function, but candles, water, and flowers make compatible offerings alongside essential oils.

You can also offer objects that have a special significance to you, such as a figure of Christ or Buddha, or whatever you wish to be blessed. Natural objects that reflect the transitory nature of existence, a fall leaf perhaps, also make good offerings. You might like to cover the shelf or table with a beautiful cloth before placing your offerings.

It is important to keep your altar clean and replace the offerings every day, or every time you meditate or perform a ritual. These preliminaries are an integral and important aspect of spiritual practice and should not be neglected. This ritual cleaning and renewing of offerings allow your altar to reflect your own needs and moods; indeed you offer part of yourself in your spiritual practice.

Essential oil burners

Most essential oil burners are ceramic and have space for a night-light candle below a bowl. The oils burn better if they are floated on top of water. Choose the most beautiful burner to place on your altar, and carefully select where you wish to position it.

When you ritually prepare your burner to offer the fragrance of essential oils, reflect that this offering incorporates all the elements. The clay of the ceramic is earth, the night-light is fire, the water is itself, and the vapor of the oils is diffused in air. In some spiritual and alchemical traditions there is also ether, and the vapor of the oils represents this subtle energy winging its way to the heavens as a divine offering.

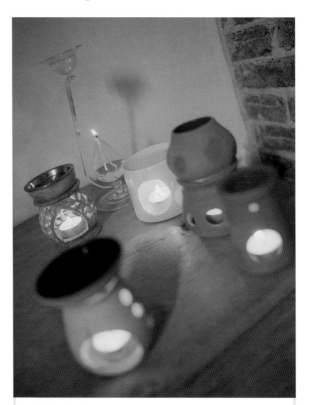

Essential oil burners
There is a wide range of essential oil burners available. Choose one that you feel is appropriate for spiritual practice, that combines esthetic and practical qualities.

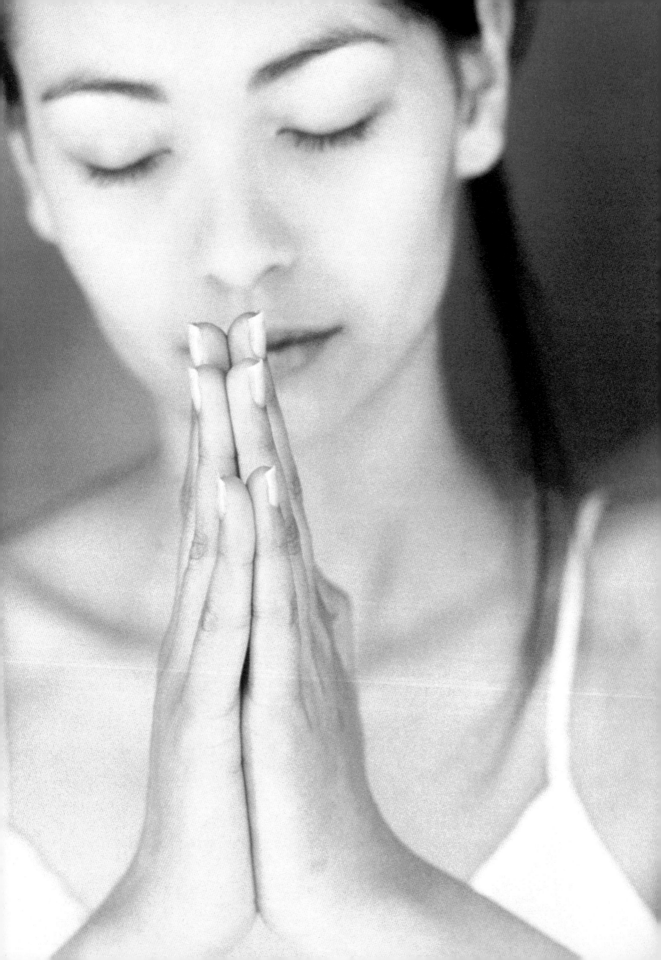

Meditation:
Heaven's Scents

When we meditate we not only discover inner peace and happiness, but we also feel better because meditation promotes healing and good health. On a deeper level, we gain insights into the meaning of being alive, here and now and from moment to moment, which is liberating and joyful.

transform

depths

"Meditation has an extraordinary power: the power to transform our lives. It is a way of finding direct access to the depths of ourselves, and to understanding our inner lives. It gives us the potential to transform misery, conflict, and neurosis. Through meditation we attend to feelings, **thoughts**, perceptions, body, health, energy, awareness, and range of experiences. Meditation can be applied to every single moment of the day."

CHRISTOPHER TITMUSS: *THE POWER OF MEDITATION*

What is Meditation?

"[Meditation] sharpens and intensifies our powers of direct perception: it gives us eyes to see into the true nature of things."

JOHN SNELLING: *THE BUDDHIST HANDBOOK*

MEDITATION HELPS US WAKE UP TO BEING IN the here-and-now, letting go of past memories and future fantasies. We become aware of the continuous stream of thoughts as they arise in our mind as simply thoughts; we do not engage with them. This state of bare awareness helps us let go of our usual ego-centered preoccupations—in other words to simply be.

Meditation is also called contemplation in some traditions, and there are different meditation practices, though they share similar goals. Meditation is part of all the great religions of the world, but you do not have to be religious or follow a particular religion to meditate, though this can be useful. However, a meditation teacher is indispensable. Meditation itself is a spiritual practice in the sense that it puts us in touch with our inner life and makes us realize our interdependence with all life.

There are three main forms of meditation, which will be explained with instructions. These are mindful awareness meditation, insight meditation, and visualization meditation. In practice they are often alternated, and mindful awareness meditation is always practiced first in order to quieten the mind. All meditations make you aware of your breathing, and often the breath is the focus of attention.

Meditation

All major religions include meditation or contemplation practices. Here, a saddhu or Indian holy man meditates according to the Hindu tradition, sitting in the traditional cross-legged posture.

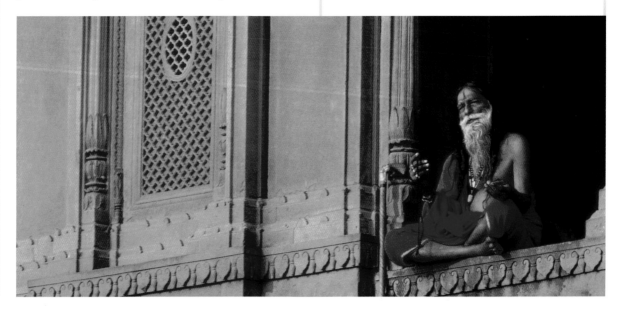

The importance of the breath

Awareness of breathing is realizing you are alive in the here-and-now. Our lives are fragile and impermanent, and if we did not breathe for a few moments we would die. The difference between life and death hangs on a breath. Breathing is not something we do; it is involuntary and our bodies know how to breathe without our conscious control.

Becoming aware of your breathing also allows you to realize your interdependence with your environment; you inhale and exhale air from your surroundings. Without the natural world changing carbon dioxide into oxygen, the air we breathe would not sustain us. Thus, interdependence extends beyond our immediate environment to embrace the world.

Meditation with essential oils adds another dimension to awareness of the breath, as we breathe in diffused aromatic particles along with air. Instead of just thinking "oh that smells nice," we can learn to feel how the oils affect our minds, moods,

"There is an excess in spiritual searching that is profound ignorance. Let that ignorance be our teacher! The friend breathes into one who has no breath."

RUMI

and bodies. We can visualize the journey of the aromatic molecules from the nose to the lungs to the bloodstream and eventually to all the different parts of the body.

This awareness of mind and body in the present moment is the aim of meditation. Of course, our minds wander all the time—especially when we first start—but if we meditate regularly and often, gradually we notice that we spend less time following our thoughts as we habitually do and discover a state of simply being.

Meditation is a useful practice, because it lessens our neurotic self-obsessions and allows us to find peace and happiness. The meditative state is healing and refreshing; it brings clarity and insight and allows our intuitive faculties to come through. We can use essential oils with meditation to connect with our own gods and spiritual wisdom, and to find inner peace and harmony.

Breathing

Awareness of the breath is fundamental to meditation. Vaporizing essential oils while meditating can help awareness of breathing, as well as influence mood and emotions.

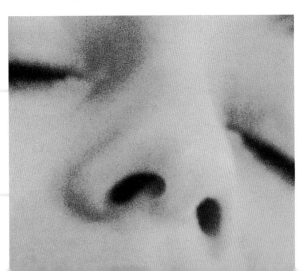

The Different Traditions of Meditation

"I have decided to go
Where springs not fail,
To fields where flies no sharp
*   and sided hail*
And a few lilies blow.
And I have asked to be
Where no storms come,
Where the green swell is in
*   the havens dumb,*
And out of the swing of the sea."
GERARD MANLEY HOPKINS

THIS BEAUTIFUL POEM CALLED *HEAVEN-HAVEN* commemorates a Christian nun taking the veil and captures the quality of a life dedicated to meditation and prayer. Christianity had a well developed esoteric aspect until the advent of the Council of Nicaea in 325CE, after which religious and secular power were gradually combined. The religious hierarchy insisted the link with God required a priest, so solitary meditation was discouraged.

Nonetheless, Christian meditation was kept alive by those who practiced secretly, and informally in monasteries and nunneries by spiritual individuals. Many Christians drawn to pray in times of crisis find meditation in silent communication with God. Christian retreats dedicated to silent worship are full of people in inner prayer and contemplation—states which have much in common with meditation.

Influence from the East

In the last few decades, Judaism and Islam from the Middle East and Hinduism and Buddhism from India and the Far East have become increasingly popular in the West. This interest developed partly from the increased number of people traveling and encountering foreign religions—alongside Easterners moving West—but also from dissatisfaction with materialism and the need to find alternative religious expression.

As a result it is now relatively easy to find Hindu ashrams (religious communities), Sufi groups, and Buddhist organizations in most Western countries. Much of the appeal of these spiritual traditions is their emphasis on the practice of meditation, although the exotic culture and the theology are of interest, too. The simplicity of an Asian spiritual lifestyle lends itself ideally to the practice of meditation.

Perhaps the most easily accessible of these traditions in the modern world is Buddhism, which has been described as the fastest growing religion in the West. The Dalai Lama, a Tibetan Buddhist monk, has wide international appeal, and his message of peace and compassion inspires many people to seek for themselves the essence of the Buddhist teachings.

People practicing meditation in the various spiritual traditions appear differently. Sufi meditation includes the practice of whirling (spinning around in a tight circle, which becomes the focus of attention). A Hindu saddhu meditating by the River Ganges wears sandalwood paste and a lot of ashes, but very little else. A Zen Buddhist monk in gray robes sits bolt upright facing the wall. In a Christian retreat a woman silently repeats her mantra, quietly sitting.

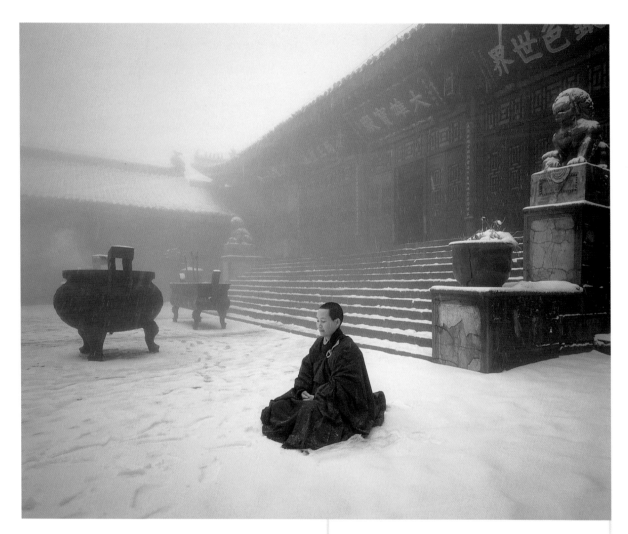

All these people share in common a spiritual yearning for inner peace and tranquillity. Though they may look different, their practices are similar, and these traditions are all familiar with burning incense and aromatics as offerings, and to facilitate communion with God. They may make meditation look difficult or unfamiliar, but meditation is accessible to everyone here and now.

Mental concentration

This Chinese Zen monk meditates in the snow, showing the depth of his concentration, at the Jinding (or Golden Summit) Temple, Sichuan Province. He develops his mental concentration to the point where he no longer feels cold.

How is Meditation Useful Today?

*"[Meditation] sharpens
and intensifies our powers
of direct perception:
it gives us eyes
to see into the true
nature of things."*

JOHN SNELLING: *A BUDDHIST HANDBOOK*

A COMMON COMPLAINT FOR MOST OF US IS that we just don't have enough time to do all the things we want to in our hectic lives. For many people five days a week is dominated by work at their job, and the weekend by work on the house and garden. Evenings tend to be spent socializing or slumped in front of the television. On the annual vacation some people even set themselves sightseeing agendas that are as demanding as any work schedule. The problem is that we don't know how to rest and relax properly.

This lifestyle also neglects the deeper side of life and spiritual issues. We might talk about meaningful things occasionally, perhaps when we are inspired by someone's contribution to resolving conflict peacefully, but we rarely make an effort ourselves. Yet we experience the lack of inner strength and peace as an unconscious malaise; we can't quite explain what we are missing.

Meditation is an invaluable resource to improve the quality of our lives. You might think finding fifteen minutes a day to meditate would increase the pressure of fulfilling your schedule, but if you willingly choose to do this you will find the benefits immeasurable. Christopher Titmuss describes meditation as an alternative to living the hectic and mind-numbing life described above. You can discover this for yourself by simply making the choice to meditate regularly.

A lifestyle including regular meditation helps heal the existential pain and dilemmas we often repress. It helps us realize that life just *is*; we cannot control what happens, but accepting this is liberating.

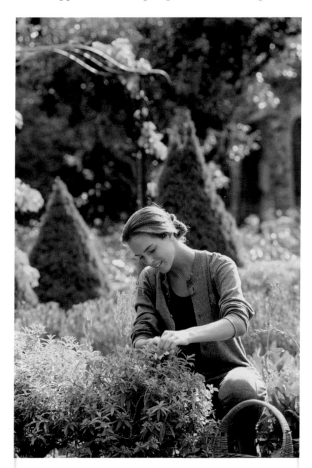

Gardening

Working in the garden can be an informal meditation that brings us closer to Nature, if we focus on being in the garden and not think about the past or future or fantasize.

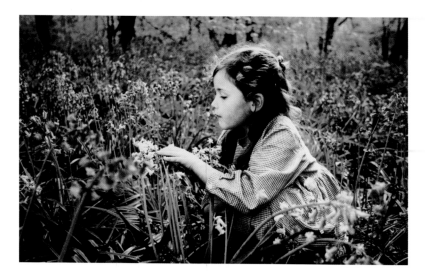

Wonder
This little girl is full of wonder at the beauties of Nature in a bluebell wood. Meditation helps us rediscover the wonder of childhood that we tend to lose as we grow older.

The benefits of meditation

There are many benefits of meditation. My favorite is the joy of not doing anything, just being aware of being alive. This leads to less stress, more energy, and the experience of an inner life. Meditation helps you to resolve difficult problems by bringing clarity and calm. Often when we feel angry we respond immediately in an aggressive way. If we quietly analyze the problem, we can find a way to respond that alleviates rather than aggravates the situation.

Although meditation is a personal, inner experience it makes you feel more open to others by realizing other people have the same feelings, fears, hopes, and inadequacies that you experience. Meditating is taking care of an important part of yourself, and when this is nurtured you are able to care for others more authentically. Your attention becomes more focused through meditation, so you find you can listen to other people without feeling the need to interject your own experiences.

Meditation brings self-knowledge and helps us to discover love, compassion, and an inner wisdom. We often think of knowledge as "out there" in books and training courses—which is partly true—but we all have vast, untapped resources inside as well. This is intuition, and meditation allows this quality to become more conscious. We feel less fragmented, more whole, as a result.

Through meditation we realize what is important in life, and the fragile impermanent nature of it, so we naturally reflect on deeper issues. This makes us less selfish, more generous, more open and loving toward ourselves and others. We see ourselves as part of the picture, not the center of the world. When our self-concern lessens, we experience peace and calm. We stop being self-obsessed and find the wonder in life and in Nature, which we see through the eyes of children. We stop trying to control events so rigidly, and let life flow naturally through both difficulties and joys.

Preparation for Meditation

"Try to experience some moments of thoughtlessness, some kind of empty feeling like the deep ocean; waves on the surface come and go in the same way that our thoughts arise and pass away, but we do not have to follow them."

THE DALAI LAMA: *SECULAR MEDITATION*

BOTH THE TIME OF DAY AND THE PLACE IN WHICH you meditate should be consistent so that you can form a familiar, comfortable habit. The benefits of meditation are experienced over time, so developing a daily meditation practice is ideal. When you start meditating, your enthusiasm must be balanced with determination to keep going.

Your daily meditation should be no longer than ten to fifteen minutes. This will seem quite long if you have not meditated before. A meditation teacher will help enormously with any questions, doubts, or concerns you may have, and attending a meditation center to meditate with others is inspiring.

You will be meditating using essential oils, so it is best to sit in front of your altar with an essential oil burner on it. If you choose not to make an altar, then a quiet place with space for your burner is fine. It is important to feel comfortable; but whether you sit on a cushion on the floor, kneel with a meditation stool, or sit on a chair is a personal choice.

Try to select a time of day for your meditation practice that you can keep to. Most people find either early morning or some time in the evening the easiest. Morning is good, because the mind is fresh and clear, and also you are rested from a night's sleep. Meditating first thing is a lovely way to start the day, but if you feel that your mind will be distracted by worrying about work, or being late, then evening is better.

After a day's work when you come through the door you probably feel tired and the last thing you want is to do something else. However, meditation is being not doing and is calming and restful, so this is a good time. If you have children or other commitments, you may find just before going to bed suits you better, but you need to be careful not to fall asleep! Meditating at this time allows you to find peace and tranquillity after the activities of the day and promotes a good night's sleep.

Posture

The most important aspect of any meditation posture is to keep the back straight. If you like to sit on a meditation cushion, position it to support the back balanced on the pelvis with the legs crossed in front. You could try a meditation stool, on which you sit with your legs tucked underneath. An alternative is a chair, but it is important to sit straight without using the back rest and with both feet on the ground.

Experiment to find which posture suits you best, always remembering to keep a straight back. This allows the energy in the body to flow freely, and though it may seem a little rigid at first it is in fact the most comfortable way to sit. Incline the head slightly forward, and keep your eyes half-open, looking down or loosely shut. Your arms should be relaxed with the hands gently folded in your lap, and the whole posture should be relaxed and free from tension. Body and mind rely on each other, and a good posture will help your meditation go well.

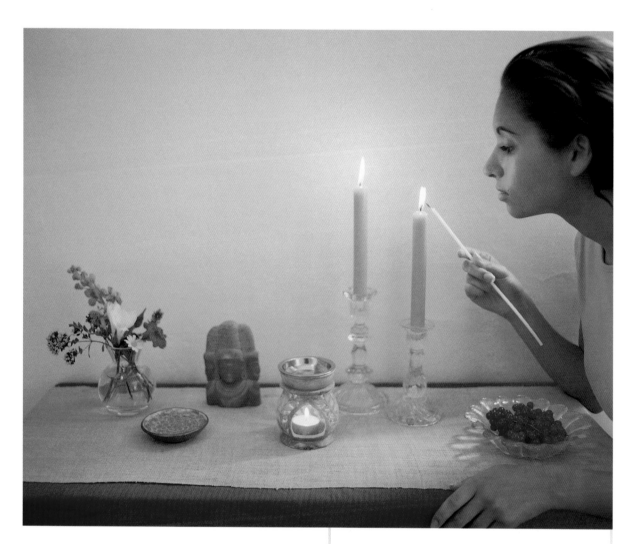

When discomfort arises, try not to fidget or change position immediately; you should simply notice the sensations in your body and try not to react. You may well find that the discomfort will pass on its own. If the discomfort you experience becomes painful, then gently shift your position, but try to learn to sit still for the duration of your meditation.

Preparation

Preparing your altar before you sit to meditate also prepares your inner self. Focus your mind clearly on what you are doing and the motivation for meditation as you light candles, arrange flowers, and prepare the essential oil burner.

Meditating with Essential Oils

"When the soul approaches the mysteries; when it tries to rally to the great spiritual principles, the perfumes are there. The odor of incense and roses fills the temples and churches of every religion in the world."

MARGUERITE MAURY: *MARGUERITE MAURY'S GUIDE TO AROMATHERAPY*

ESSENTIAL OIL BURNERS ARE POTTERY OR CERAMIC and have a lower space for a night-light candle and an upper bowl for water, on top of which is floated between ten and fifteen drops of essential oil. The heat from the candle warms the water and the essential oils evaporate along with steam. Electric diffusers and light bulb rings are also available, but the natural and ritualistic style of using burners makes them most appropriate for use on an altar.

To prepare the burner before your meditation, decide which oil or blend of oils you are going to use. This requires analyzing how you feel and what you wish to gain from the meditation. For example, you may feel tired and want to feel refreshed after your meditation session, so you would choose a mentally stimulating oil such as basil or rosemary and an uplifting oil such as bergamot, rosewood, or mandarin.

Check if there is any emotional disturbance, so if you also feel you've had a long, tough day you could add a soothing, nurturing oil such as benzoin, ylang ylang, or rose. Every blend is a unique creation, so allow your intuition to come into play; your unconscious mind and your body may have some good ideas too.

Using three oils creates an effective synergy, but do a sniff test first and add the oils drop by drop to obtain the right proportions. Fill the bowl about three-quarters full of water and float the essential oils on top. Then light the candle underneath. Some designs make the water heat slowly, which gives you time to make some offerings on your altar.

Alternatively, you can start your meditation session and allow the aroma of the oils to arise gradually. If you are short of time and want to smell the oils quickly, you could pour hot or near-boiling water in the bowl, then add the drops of essential oil very carefully.

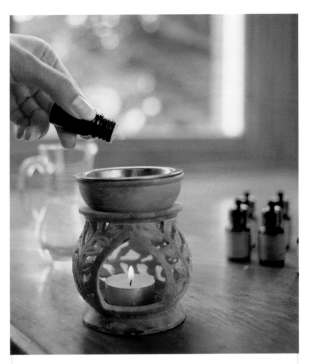

Oil burners

Essential oil burners are often esthetically pleasing. Once placed on your altar they become part of the sacred space and the offerings, so it is best to choose an attractive one.

> *"Certain essential oils such as sandalwood, jasmine or rose make excellent perfumes dabbed neat on the skin."*
>
> **JULIA LAWLESS:**
> ***THE ENCYCLOPEDIA OF ESSENTIAL OILS***

Room sprays and anointing

Burners produce a powerful aroma, because once the water is hot the oils diffuse quickly. If a more subtle effect is preferred on occasion, then you can use a room spray. Purchase an unused perfume spray bottle, or you can use one that has held pure flower waters, also called hydrosols or hydrolats. Half-fill it with water and then add your choice of essential oils. Essential oils do not dissolve in water, so they will float on the top, but a vigorous shake will disperse them temporarily in the water, and then you can spray the mixture into the room.

Anointing can be used in meditation and in ritual. There may be times, for example when you are practicing walking meditation or are traveling when you don't have a burner with you; or sometimes you may prefer to wear essential oils. This is also the most economical way of using the expensive absolutes, and they make delightful fragrances.

However, care must be taken when using essential oils neat on the skin, and certain oils should be avoided such as the citrus oils, which are photosensitizing and could discolor your skin if used in sunlight. Spices can be skin irritants, so avoid these, too. The florals and absolutes as well as frankincense, sandalwood, and rosewood are fine. Use only one or two drops and on a small area, preferably behind your ears or the inside of your wrist. Although unlikely, if you do experience any irritation or redness, you should simply wash the oils off your skin.

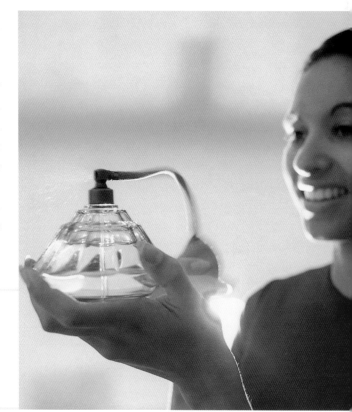

Room sprays

Room sprays are an effective, though less powerful, alternative method to diffuse the oils into the room. An unused perfume bottle is suitable for essential oils because it is uncontaminated by perfume.

Meditating Regularly and Changing the Oils

"Mindfulness is essential for successful meditation; and in our day-to-day lives it keeps us centered, alert and conscientious, helping us know what is happening in our mind as it happens and thus to deal skilfully with problems."

KATHLEEN MCDONALD: *HOW TO MEDITATE*

YOU NEED TO MEDITATE REGULARLY AND OFTEN— ideally once a day—to appreciate fully the benefits of meditation. In this way it becomes a way of life or being, rather than an activity you occasionally do. If you cannot manage daily, meditating on alternate days, or a few times a week, maintains the flow and rhythm. You should not force yourself to meditate; it should be a pleasant break from mundane life, so try to find a balance of discipline and enjoyment.

You do not need a specific reason to meditate; meditating simply to enhance life and to develop inner peace is sufficient motivation. When troublesome moods and issues arise, then specific meditations to deal with these can be practiced alongside a general meditation practice. Regular meditation can resolve problems more effectively and help you to see the consequences of your actions, before you react without thinking.

When you meditate regularly with essential oils you have to be careful not to fall into the habit of using the same oils repeatedly. There are many different essential oils and thousands of combinations, plus variations by changing the proportions, so there is no excuse for using the same oil or blend continuously! Don't just use essential oils you think are holy or religious; any oil can provide a spiritual experience. Stay bold, and experiment so that each meditation has a special blend; it will keep the experience fresh and alive each time you meditate.

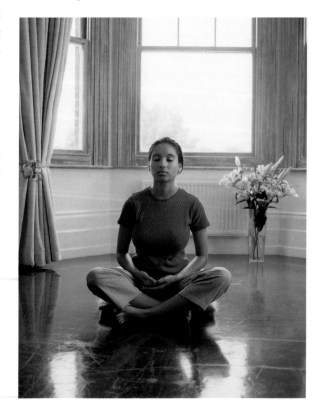

Meditation

Meditation is a powerful tool for self-discovery, an internal process of becoming familiar with the mind and thought processes. This inner knowing helps us let go of our neurotic obsessions and find inner tranquillity.

The importance of changing the oils

As any aromatherapist will tell you, it is important to change the essential oils you use frequently. This is because the body becomes accustomed to a particular oil or blend of oils, and then they work less effectively. Both ourselves and the oils are organic, living, changing beings, and we adapt quickly to substances that affect us. This is also why we get "bored" if we eat the same food, use the same shampoo, toothpaste, or deodorant all the time; we need diversity for a rich experience of life.

As you experiment and play with the oils you will notice that you have definite favorites, as well as oils you don't like. Stay with the process of exploration; after some time you will discover new favorites, go off old ones, and decide you really like an oil you detested at the beginning. Our minds and bodies instinctively know what we need beyond our intellectual ideas of what we consciously think we need. So we should include all our reactions when choosing the oils we are going to use for meditation. Remember, too, that you are changing all the time in subtle ways, and that what you need at any time will reflect these subtle changes.

It is also important not to impose limits on your-self according to what you have read or been told. If, for example, you are searching for essential oils to

"The compelling power of odors on the psyche has been recognized since the very earliest times."

**ROBERT TISSERAND:
THE ART OF
AROMATHERAPY**

use in meditation, and you have analyzed how you feel and are making an appropriate selection accordingly, but something just doesn't feel right, then pause. Maybe you are suppressing some emotion that needs to be expressed. On the other hand, maybe your mind and body continuum requires something you hadn't considered.

In cases such as these let your nose be a guide, and let your intuition draw you to whatever essential oils and combinations it wants to. The oils that you choose by smell and intuition can tell you something about what is going on inside you, so you can use this information in your meditation to get in touch with your deepest feelings. In this way meditation with essential oils becomes a powerful tool for self-discovery.

Meditation is like spring cleaning the mind; we want peace and clarity, but we have to recognize and clean away dust and cobwebs first. Meditating with appropriate essential oils on each occasion helps lessen the intensity of our greatest recurring fears as we learn to see them as impermanent and not integral to our mind.

With experience you will become familiar with your inner life through regular meditation. This self-awareness helps you select the essential oils that will bring the greatest benefit to each meditation session.

Mindful Awareness Meditation

"The most important thing is not to set ambitious goals or strive for results—that is more likely to frustrate rather than hasten the development of concentration—but to simply perform the practice patiently and aim first and foremost at remaining aware of what is going on in the Now."

JOHN SNELLING: *A BUDDHIST HANDBOOK*

MINDFUL AWARENESS MEDITATION IS WHERE we start from. We remain largely unaware of the nature of our mind if we don't meditate, and when we first begin meditation it seems as if the mind is full of racing thoughts that were not there before. However, this is an illusion; because we usually just indulge and follow our thoughts and feelings, we never realize how they fully occupy our mind.

When you notice the contents of your mind as you begin meditating, it is normal to feel that you can't do it, that you will never be able to sit quietly and just be without thinking. Though meditation aims for this bare awareness, in practice it is rarely achieved unless you dedicate much of your life to meditation. Mindful awareness meditation is simply noting thoughts and feelings as they arise in the mind, not suppressing or indulging them, but choosing to let them go.

You don't want to be distracted by anything during your meditation session, so remember to put on your answerphone, or pull out the telephone connection. You also don't want to be preoccupied with the time, so when you start set an alarm clock to ring after the fifteen minutes are up. If you hear any sound during your meditation session, ignore it. Think of it as noise and let it go. You have chosen to meditate for this time; this is what is important.

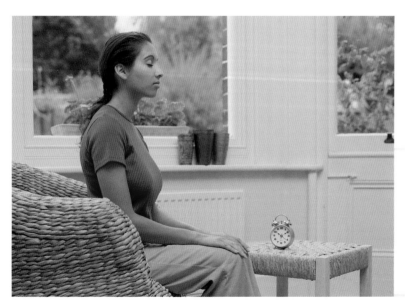

Mindful awareness

When we practice mindful awareness meditation, frustration often arises. The meditation seems very simple, but it can be difficult in practice. If you feel frustrated, try to regard that feeling as just another thought and let it go.

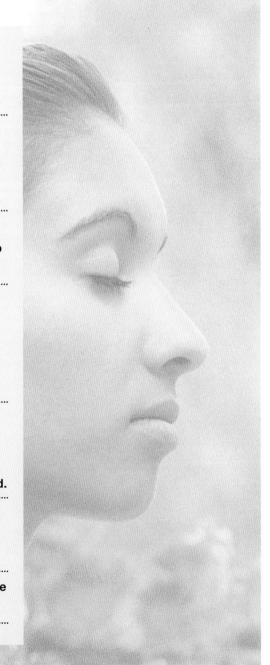

Mindful Awareness Meditation

Prepare your burner, make offerings, and resolve to meditate for fifteen minutes without giving up.

Sit in the meditation posture you have selected, and bring your attention to your breathing. Don't try to breathe any differently—just be aware of the sensation of the breath entering and leaving your body.

Notice all the different thoughts, fantasies, memories, and feelings in your mind, and resolve to let them all go and simply watch your breath.

When your mind wanders, don't be hard on yourself; this is what it normally does, and it will take time and effort to change it. Simply return your attention to the breath, and be aware of breathing in the essential oils as you inhale, but don't think about them.

Even if your mind seems to race furiously it doesn't matter. Being aware of the here-and-now through your breathing is what counts; meditation is not a competition to see how quickly you can calm your mind.

Don't be tempted by a wonderful idea or thought; you have chosen to meditate for fifteen minutes, and you can think all your thoughts afterward.

When you finish meditating, try to take the quality of the feeling with you when you move into your daily life.

Mindful Awareness Meditation for Anger

"The effect of some odours on the emotions are quite strong. The writer, working with odorous materials for more than twenty years, long ago noticed that ... ylang ylang oil soothes and inhibits anger born of frustration."

R.W. MONCRIEFF: *ODOURS*

UNDERSTANDING THE CAUSES OF ANGER HELPS US to transform the energy and restore harmony. Anger is hot, sudden, red, overwhelming, and violent. It can have a devastating effect on others and yourself, so it is worth the effort to investigate how anger arises.

Anger is not simply emotional; it is mental and physical too, as we can see from the interrelationship between these different aspects of ourselves. We often describe angry people with the words "their blood was up," and those with high blood pressure are often quick to anger. Blood is also purified by the liver, which is associated with anger, and we still use the old expression "liverish" to describe irritability. Thus we can see the link between alcohol and anger.

Essential oils

Several essential oils are useful in dealing with anger and are cooling, calming, and sedative. These include ylang ylang, benzoin, melissa, chamomile, and rose. Irritability is also helped by lavender, marjoram, cypress, frankincense, and sandalwood.

One of the German chamomiles is called blue chamomile, and the cooling effect of the blue helps calm the red heat of anger. Blue chamomile contains aszulene, which gives the blue tinge, and as well as calming the emotions it also soothes itchy skin and a racing mind.

Anger is a complex emotion and may have different subtle interrelated causes. We tend to get angry as a reaction, which we usually put down to some external cause. However, often we react angrily because of lack of self-confidence, insecurity, and feelings of being hurt, or hormonal causes such as premenstrual syndrome.

So, when we are choosing essential oils for a meditation on calming anger, we need to reflect on our mind, body, emotions, and spirit. For example, if we feel angry when we are asked to do something we find challenging, we may also be feeling insecure and lacking in confidence. Thus we choose oils to reflect the full complexity of how we are feeling.

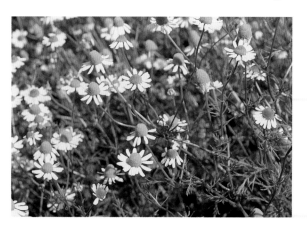

Chamomile

Chamomile is a useful essential oil to vaporize with a mindful awareness meditation for anger. The gentle but penetrating fragrance of chamomile soothes troubled emotions and helps calm an agitated mind.

Meditation on Anger

Prepare the oil burner with the oils you have selected.

Start by watching your breath. Notice if your anger has made your breathing quicker and more shallow. If so, take a few long, slow, deep breaths, experiencing the smell of the oils, and then resume watching your breath.

Allow your feelings of anger, hurt, or frustration to simply be present. Try not to get involved in them, but acknowledge them and attempt to let them go.

If your feelings intensify and you get drawn in, return your attention to your breathing.

Feel the vaporized oils entering your nose, and, if you like, visualize them traveling around your body. Imagine them softening your breathing and opening your heart.

Don't judge yourself for feeling angry, or try to suppress it. Breathe into the anger and let it calm down.

Continue watching your breath and enjoying the sensation of the oils.

"Anger cannot be overcome with anger. If a person shows anger to you, and you respond with anger, the result is disastrous. In contrast, if you control the anger and show opposite attitudes—compassion, tolerance, and patience—then not only do you yourself remain in peace, but the other's anger will gradually diminish."

DALAI LAMA:
KINDNESS, CLARITY & INSIGHT

Insight Meditation

"The practice of mindful awareness is a first step in the direction of inner freedom... Such stillness, though, is not an end in itself. It serves as a platform from which to observe more clearly what is taking place within us."

STEPHEN BATCHELOR:
THE AWAKENING OF THE WEST

WHEN YOU HAVE ACHIEVED SOME CALM AND clarity in your mind through practicing mindful awareness meditation, it is natural to wish to inquire into all these distracting thoughts and feelings that continuously arise in your mind. You have probably made the unsettling discovery that you are not in control of what or how you think. This is where insight meditation is useful.

Once the mind is able to focus clearly through practicing mindful awareness meditation, it is time to look deeply at what appears in the mind and analyze it. This scrutiny of our thoughts and feelings is not comfortable; we may all have thoughts and fantasies we would rather not admit to. However, it is natural for these to arise, and it is important not to judge yourself or try to suppress anything.

Usually when we think thoughts and experience feelings, we unquestioningly identify with them. Insight meditation gives us some distance. You learn to see them as just thoughts and feelings that happened to pop into your mind rather than as part of yourself. You may notice that these contents of the mind are fleeting and insubstantial.

Through analysis of our thoughts and feelings we realize that not only are they temporary, they do not bring much happiness, and we notice a lot of dissatisfaction. This can lead to the realization that true happiness lies beyond individual feelings and thoughts. Mindfully watching all the contents of our mind simply flow past without identifying with or indulging them in any way can eventually bring true inner peace. Be aware that when you start insight meditation, old repressed memories tend to surface, and these can be painful.

It is important not to give up at this stage, and as and when disturbing thoughts and painful memories arise give them space, but do not identify with them. They will disappear from consciousness when they are ready.

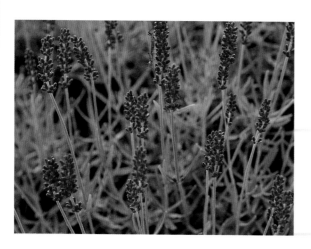

Lavender

Lavender helps calm the mind, together with mindful awareness of breathing meditation, and helps develop the focus and clarity necessary for insight meditation.

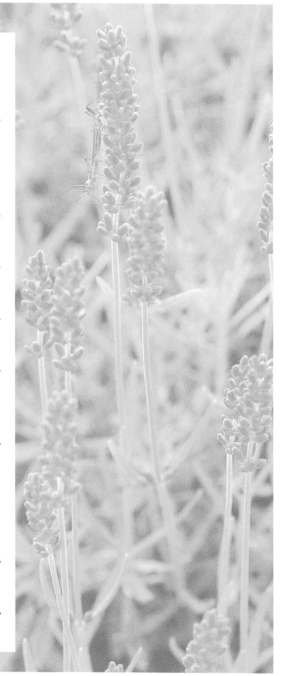

Insight Meditation

Prepare your burner with the essential oils you have chosen for this meditation session.

Sit comfortably in your meditation posture and spend a few minutes observing your breath in mindful awareness meditation to calm your mind and strengthen your concentration.

Be aware of your thoughts and feelings as they come and go.

Bring your attention to whatever arises and concentrate strongly on it.

Go beyond a superficial look. Analyze your thoughts and feelings as they arise.

When you notice you have become distracted, bring your attention back to the breath for a few minutes, until your mind is clear and calm again.

If you become upset, remember these thoughts, feelings, and memories are impermanent; they arise and pass in the same way as all others. Remember the oils you are burning, and breathe in deeply to gain the benefit.

Spend the last few minutes of your meditation session watching the breath.

Insight Meditation for Frustrated Desire

"Sometimes we experience a tremendous desire for something. This wanting can become a real pressure in our minds. We feel that we will not have any peace of mind unless we get what we want. This can lead to unhappiness and disappointment."

CHRISTOPHER TITMUSS:
THE POWER OF MEDITATION

WE ALL HAVE LOTS OF DESIRES. IF WE THINK BACK, we have always had a lot of desires; some remain unfulfilled, but as we change over time, often we no longer crave what we once wanted so much. Some unfulfilled desires may remain with us for a long time, and we still crave the object of this desire.

What does this tell us about the nature of desire? Most important, it tells us that desire usually makes us unhappy. Consequently, letting go of wanting objects, relationships, and so on is more likely to bring us happiness. Even if we experience happiness because a cherished desire is realized, this passes quickly and we no longer feel happy when we have got what we wanted. Usually we start wanting something else immediately!

If we weigh up the brief happiness from fulfilling a desire against the prevalence of dissatisfaction from unfulfilled desire, we see that desire does not bring a true and lasting happiness. Insight meditation helps us let go of desire by analyzing the objects of desire. In this way we realize that however many of our desires are fulfilled, the mind will continue to want other things.

For example, you might crave wealth in the mistaken belief that it will bring you happiness. Imagine that you suddenly acquire a great deal of money. Of course you are thrilled for a short while. Then you worry about how much to spend on the dream vacation, car, and so on. You buy a fantastic house, and fill it with beautiful objects, but worry about security. You become suspicious that your friends are envious of your good fortune, and you see them less. One day you wake up, lonely in a dream house that no longer has the same appeal. Were you perhaps happier before?

Insight meditation helps us to analyze our desires, so we can see which are realistically achievable. This helps us let go of a theoretical future happiness and appreciate what we have here and now.

Essential oils

We can use oils that are mentally stimulating and balancing, such as basil, rosemary, and geranium. We also need to include an essential oil that will help us to soften our firmly held beliefs. Rose and benzoin open and soften our hearts, and help us not to feel jealous.

Bergamot, mandarin, and orange assist us to find happiness in the present moment. There are many antidepressant oils, and those best suited to frustration include chamomile, linden blossom, lavender, and clary sage.

Including an oil that facilitates introspection, helps you to penetrate deeply into your feelings, and perhaps learn from past experiences. These oils include myrrh, frankincense, narcissus, and violet leaf.

Meditation for Frustrated Desire

Select your oils and prepare your burner. Spend a few minutes in mindful awareness meditation.

Reflect on your desires and focus firmly on whichever manifests most strongly. Analyze the nature of this desire. Does it have any inherent features that can guarantee you lasting happiness?

Remember realizing a cherished desire. How long was it before the happiness faded and was replaced by a desire for something else?

If your mind wanders into desire itself, return your attention to your breath. Feel the oils entering your body and experience their effect.

Finish the meditation session with awareness of your breath and oils, and feel whether this brings you happiness now.

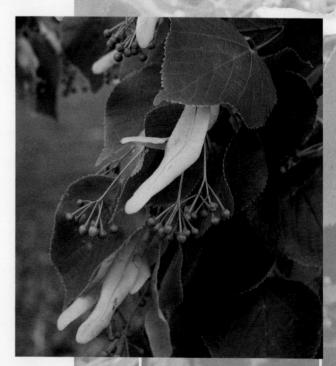

Linden blossom

The sweet, voluptuous fragrance of linden blossom helps us feel happy in the here-and-now, and so it lessens the frustration of desire.

Walking Meditation

"Formal walking meditation is a form of contemplative expression. This means that we walk unusually slowly… The act of walking matters more than the preoccupation with destination or where we are coming from."

CHRISTOPHER TITMUSS:
THE POWER OF MEDITATION

WALKING MEDITATION IS AN ALTERNATIVE posture, rather than a different form of meditation. So we can do mindful awareness, insight, or visualization meditations while engaged in walking meditation. It has many benefits and combines well with sitting meditation if you wish to meditate for a longer time. Walking meditation has been practiced by Christians and Buddhists for centuries. It still has great appeal, especially to those with a hectic lifestyle.

If you find it painful or difficult to sit in meditation, then walking meditation is a good alternative, though it is best to do a short sitting meditation session first. Once you have gained some meditation experience, you may well wish to lengthen your meditations. Alternating between sitting and walking sessions of fifteen minutes each gives you the opportunity to know when you have done enough. Walking meditation keeps the flow of meditating while allowing your body to stretch tired or cramped muscles and joints.

Walking meditation is done in a short straight line, with a pause at the end when you turn around and retrace your steps. Although it can be done indoors, this is a wonderful opportunity to meditate in Nature and feel the connection with all life. You have to remember not to become distracted by the beauty of flowers or birdsong, simply to appreciate and acknowledge them without getting drawn in.

Using essential oils for walking meditation is easy. If you are doing walking meditation inside, use your burner as with sitting meditation. If you are outside, use the anointing method. If you wish to use oils that are not safe on the skin, drop the oils onto a tissue and tuck it in a top pocket or similarly close to your nose so you can access the aroma. Without the heat of the burner or warmth of your skin, the oils diffuse less pungently, so you can use a few drops more.

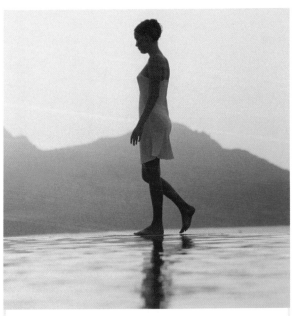

Walking meditation
Walking meditation is an alternative to sitting meditation, and when you gain experience you can practice insight or visualization meditation together with walking meditation.

Walking Meditation

Prepare your burner, anointing, or tissue with your chosen oils. Have a clear idea of your walking path; between five and ten yards (meters) is fine. If you are in a small room you can walk around in a circle. You can pause, and turn, at the point where you began, if you like.

Stand at the beginning of the line and spend a couple of minutes focusing on your breath. Then slowly and mindfully raise one foot, move it forward, feeling all the muscles involved and place it gently down, feeling heel and toes separately as they make contact with the ground. Repeat this until you reach the end of your line, then pause, turn, pause, and retrace your steps.

While walking, fold your hands gently over your abdomen or keep them relaxed at your sides.

It is a good idea to start with mindful awareness meditation, and as well as watching your breath, extend awareness to all your body. Check that you are fully relaxed.

If you become distracted, pause in your walking and watch your breath until your concentration returns, then start mindfully walking again.

Be aware of inhaling the oils as you slowly move, and feel your connection with your environment. Be mindful not to speed up; remember you are not going anywhere.

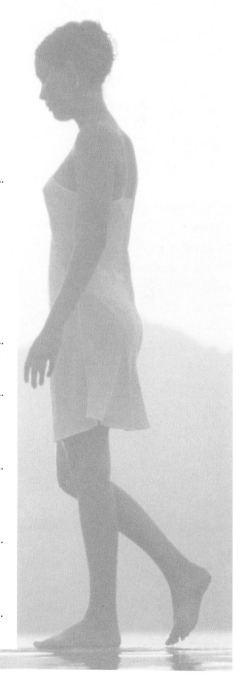

Walking Meditation for Alienation

"We need to realize that we are practicing meditation not to acquire greater powers and more possessions for ourselves, but rather to move away from the basic ego centered orientation to a new wider, more selfless one."

JOHN SNELLING: *THE BUDDHIST HANDBOOK*

OUR MODERN WORLD WITH ALL ITS technological advances and abundance of materialism can be a lonely place, and lack meaning. Many of us have to work at jobs that give us little creative or personal satisfaction. When we finish work and go home, we often read or watch television, which also ignores our inner feelings.

Neglecting our inner life can cause depression and dissatisfaction—alienation. This can cause us to become withdrawn and respond mechanically to others, or become anxious and paranoid, wondering what is wrong with us. We try to pull ourselves together, but though this may work temporarily the real problem is suppressed.

If we respond appropriately we can listen to and honor our inner life. This is a hard spiritual journey, but the inner peace and happiness we experience are worth the effort. An inspiring way to dispel alienation is by connecting with Nature by practicing walking meditation in a beautiful country place using carefully chosen essential oils.

Essential oils

Any essential oil is useful in this personal context if it resonates with you strongly. Select bottles guided by intuition, and take a quick smell from the bottle. You will know instantly if it is a good oil for you to use at this time.

However, certain essential oils are to be recommended. Angelica helps us reconnect with our spiritual side. Rosewood works in a similar way, helping us to develop and nurture neglected spiritual yearnings. Neroli and melissa allay existential anxiety, jasmine gives confidence, cedarwood strength, and patchouli endurance.

If we feel existential pain in the heart, rose, marjorma, or ylang ylang is indicated. If existential pain is in the mind, then try frankincense. If we feel confused, lemon, rosemary, juniper, cedarwood, and basil all bring clarity. Mandarin, jasmine, narcissus, or clary sage will give a slight euphoric effect, and this can help us connect with Nature's energies around us.

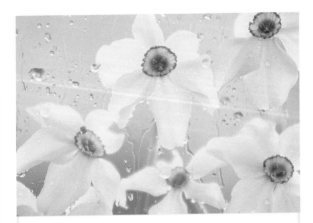

Narcissus

The slight euphoria we experience when using narcissus with walking meditation in nature helps us realize our interdependence with the natural world.

Meditation for Alienation

Find a quiet, beautiful, rural place, and time to go there alone.

Intuitively choose oils that resonate deeply with your soul. Either mix them in a little almond or other base oil and apply to your wrists and behind your ears; apply them neat, or sprinkle them on a tissue and place near your nose.

Ensure your walking path is flat and even, and that you know where to turn.

Stand for a few minutes in mindful awareness meditation starting with your breath and gradually include your whole body, then your environment and the diffused oils.

As you begin to walk slowly and mindfully, feel your interconnection with the natural world around you. It embraces you without judgment. You can be who you truly are.

If you become distracted, stand in mindful awareness meditation until your mind is focused again. At the end of your walking path pause, turn, pause, and retrace your steps.

There is no need to time this meditation; take as long as you want. When you feel it is time to finish, stand in mindful awareness meditation for a few minutes and connect with the feeling of being part of a larger whole. Take this feeling with you when you return to daily life.

Visualization Meditation

"About this mind... in truth there is nothing really wrong with it. It is intrinsically pure. Within itself it is already peaceful. Our practice is simply to see the Original Mind. So we must train the mind to know the sense impressions and not get lost in them."

AJAHN CHAH: *BODHINYANA*

VISUALIZATION MEDITATION HELPS DEVELOP focused concentration like mindful awareness meditation, but uses a visualized object instead of the breath. We also use the depth of focus developed in insight meditation to create and explore our mental image. Visualization meditation works with part of our unconscious as well, especially if we use strong archetypal images, because these symbols resonate in our psyche and help us to discover inner wisdom.

A lovely story concerns a Buddhist abbot who decided to meditate on the cross, one of the foremost symbols of Christianity. What he realized through the power of his visualization meditation was that the cross also symbolizes cutting through "I"—the main symbol of the ego. In this way a symbol from one religion became meaningful to another; the endeavor itself finding harmony between religions.

What is important is that the symbol you choose has deep meaning for you. If conventional religious symbols (such as a cross or Star of David), or Nature symbols (such as a flower, or even the whole earth) do not appeal, try to visualize what or who symbolizes a higher wisdom for you. This works best if you have a clear image; visualization meditation with hazy, abstract ideas involves a lot of work. You can vary which symbols you use over time, but—as with all meditations—regularity and frequency are important, and when you first start choose one symbol and stay with it.

Visualization meditation helps us to see things in a different way, like in the story of the Buddhist abbot. So we need to keep an open mind when we do this meditation, and after some time we will start to see our symbol in a different light. This is useful, because it shows us that there are more ways to see things than we usually believe, and that none of them is better or worse than any other. There is no right or wrong in perception, simply differences. This realization can be helpful in daily life if we disagree with someone; we can be more open to how the other person sees things.

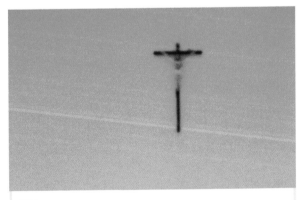

The cross

The most fundamental icon of Christianity is the cross. If you practice Christianity, or even if you just feel a close connection to Jesus, then the cross can be a powerful object of visualization meditation.

Visualization Meditation

Prepare your burner with the oils you have chosen. Bear in mind that visualization meditation can be quite difficult, so avoid oils that you find soporific.

Sit comfortably and spend a few minutes in mindful awareness meditation until your mind is clear and focused.

Bring to mind your chosen symbol. If you have a statue or picture of this image, you can use this as a meditation aid, and look at it before closing your eyes. Don't cheat and keep looking at it throughout the meditation!

Visualize the whole symbol. Try to see it in a living, vibrant form. When the image fades, concentrate on a part of it and gradually build it back up.

Be aware of your breathing and of the oils; both can help your visualization.

If your mind wanders or you feel frustrated that you can't do it, spend a few minutes in mindful awareness meditation. Then bring the image to mind again. If you find the whole image too difficult, select one part and work with that for a few meditation sessions.

Finish with watching the breath and enjoying the sensation of the oils.

Body of Light Meditation

"Remember too that visualization utilizes only the mental faculty, not the eyes. If you find that you are straining to see something, you misunderstand the technique. Relax and let the image appear from within your mind."

KATHLEEN MCDONALD: *HOW TO MEDITATE*

THIS SIMPLE VISUALIZATION MEDITATION IS for general well-being, harmony, and joy, and is a good way to start learning visualization meditation. It is not unusual to find visualization difficult, especially when you begin, so try to develop sensitivity and patience. Sometimes we have a tendency to rush into complex things, since this seems to be rewarded in our competitive, modern world. Enjoying something simple is a good antidote to the stress and tension brought about by striving for achievement.

The body of light meditation involves the whole body, so it is particularly helpful to discover areas of stress we may not have been aware of. We probably all realize when we have tense muscles in our shoulders, but it is common to hold stress in the solar plexus, for example, and remain unaware of it. Awareness is the first step to releasing tension, and the body of light meditation can help you to relax deeply and to dissipate stress you have unconsciously held on to over a long time.

Essential oils

This meditation is about promoting relaxation and happiness rather than trying to dispel negative emotion, so choose some of your current favorite oils. These have an affinity with how you feel at this time; you could say they are on the same wavelength as you.

If you have a favorite blend, this could work well, but ensure the oils are not all deep and mysterious. The body of light visualization requires predominantly light oils such as bergamot, rosewood, palmarosa, neroli, lemon, basil, mandarin, and elemi. One deeper oil can make sure you don't end up floating away altogether! A drop of rose, jasmine, linden blossom, violet leaf, patchouli, benzoin, or frankincense will provide a grounding influence.

Check your blend is harmonious by trying it out first on cotton balls to avoid being distracted by an aroma you are not quite sure you like, or by a fragrance that is too deep.

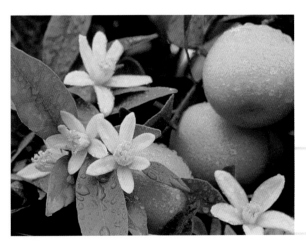

Neroli
Light oils such as neroli are especially useful for body of light meditation, because they enhance the quality of white light.

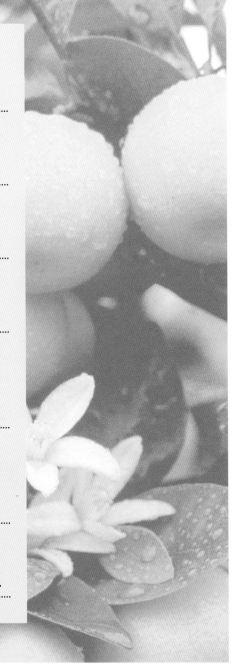

Body of Light Meditation

Prepare your burner and sit quietly in mindful awareness meditation for a few minutes until your mind is quiet.

Visualize a sphere of white light in the space above your head. Don't worry if the image is not clear, having a sense of it is enough.

Contemplate that the light represents universal love and wisdom while visualizing the image. Breathe mindfully and feel the oils entering your body.

Visualize the sphere of light descending into the top of your head and traveling down until it reaches your heart. Feel blessed by the light.

After a while visualize the light expanding to fill your whole body, and your body taking on the quality of pure white light. Imagine all negativities—depression, anger, and so on—are being transformed into love and wisdom.

Keep the body of light meditation vibrant. Feel at one with the universe, peaceful and joyful. Feel the oils flowing through your body. If distracting thoughts arise, imagine them dissolving into the white light.

When you are ready to finish, let the visualization fade, and spend a few minutes in mindful awareness meditation. Keep the sensation of relaxed happiness as you go about your life.

Group Meditation for World Peace

> *"We can never obtain peace in the world if we neglect the inner world and don't make peace with ourselves. World peace must develop out of inner peace. Without inner peace it is impossible to achieve world peace, external peace."*
>
> **DALAI LAMA: *KINDNESS, CLARITY & INSIGHT***

THE DESIRE FOR WORLD PEACE IS A COMMON vision, and group meditation is an ideal way to share such a noble aspiration. However, as we can see from the Dalai Lama's words (above), the best way to work for world peace is to work on our inner peace. Until we can maintain equanimity in both favorable and adverse circumstances and maintain our inner peace, we will continue to get caught in negative emotions.

Group meditation can be inspiring and powerful. When we feel weak, our meditation is hopeless, or our mind is distracted, then other people can listen and offer advice and support. Eventually we feel able to accept our mental distractions and carry on

meditating till our mind quietens. We can likewise offer support to others when they need it.

It is best if your group—even two people are sufficient—can meditate regularly together. You must be careful to ensure that the prime purpose of getting together is to meditate; the social aspect, however pleasant, must be secondary. A good way is to start the meditation with no conversation beforehand. You can all share your meditation experiences informally together afterward.

Essential oils

Everyone in the group must like the oils used. If there are a number of you, it might be easiest to select one essential oil each time, so you don't spend the whole meditation session discussing various exotic blends! This can be done at the end of the last session, so that you can start meditating without conversation.

The most obvious essential oil in this context is frankincense, provided that everyone in the group likes it. Rosewood is lighter and may be preferred. You should alternate the oils used, though you could stay with frankincense every other session if you like. Rose opens the heart to universal love, and mandarin is popular. However, explore different oils together, and you will find blends that bring depth and harmony to your group meditations.

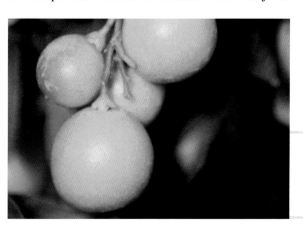

Mandarin

Mandarin is a popular oil that blends easily and, consequently, is a good choice for group meditations.

Group Meditation for World Peace

Prepare your burner with the oil or blend the group has selected. Spend a few minutes in mindful awareness meditation.

Feel the experience of meditating in a group. Check that your motivation is to develop inner peace as a contribution toward world peace.

As you watch your breath be aware of breathing in the essential oils and the quality they bring to your breathing and mind. Remember you are sharing this experience with others who have the same motivation.

Feel joyful that this occasion has arisen to share meditation with other people. Feel goodwill to everyone in your group, then allow this feeling to spread to your family and loved ones, to everyone you know, and finally to all beings everywhere. Wish that they may all find inner peace.

If you become distracted, bring your attention back to the breath. Feel the silent support of those with whom you are meditating.

At the end of the session, a designated member of the group can ring a bell—a much nicer sound than an alarm clock!

Spend a few moments enjoying inner peace in silence, then share your thoughts and experiences with each other.

Breathing Meditation According to Rumi

"There is a way between voice and presence where information flows. In disciplined silence it opens. With wandering talk it closes."

RUMI

JALALUDDIN RUMI WAS A SUFI WHO LIVED IN the thirteenth century in what was then Persia, but is now Afghanistan. Following on from his father, Rumi became a sheikh in the dervish community, giving spiritual instruction and meditating. His encounter with Shams of Tabriz, a wandering dervish, led to an extraordinary spiritual friendship that is expressed in Rumi's ecstatic, mystical poetry.

Often regarded as the greatest mystic poet of all time, Rumi's writing offers insight into the Sufi mystical tradition. His poems cut straight to the heart, tossing aside all that it is not authentic communion with God. In his poem "Only Breath," Rumi shows us that all our personas and identities are false ways of being, and that there is only a human being breathing in this moment. This makes a powerful, incisive meditation practice, and meditating with essential oils honors Rumi's sensual nature.

"The mind wants categories, but Rumi's creativity was a continuous fountaining from beyond forms and the mind, or as the Sufis say, from a mind within the mind, the *qalb*, which is a great compassionate generosity" (Coleman Barks: *The Essential Rumi*).

Choose oils that complement Rumi's direct insight, sensuality, and mystical ecstasy. A piercing oil such as basil, ginger, or rosemary will cut through intellectual theorizing to bare experience. Include something sensuous such as jasmine, ylang ylang, or sandalwood to put you in touch with your feelings, and an oil to transport your senses into the mystical realm such as narcissus, violet leaf, or angelica. You could include any oil that makes you feel ecstatic—perhaps rose, neroli, jasmine, or linden blossom.

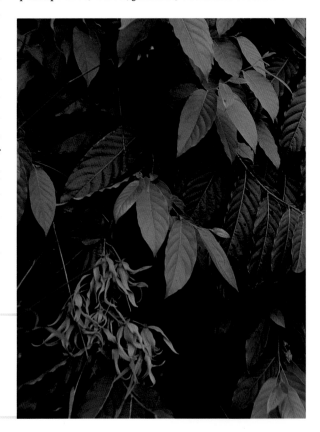

Ylang ylang
Including a sensuous essential oil such as ylang ylang in the breathing meditation according to Rumi puts you in contact with both your own and Rumi's sensual nature.

Breathing Meditation Inspired by Rumi

Prepare your burner and sit comfortably. Read Rumi's words—aloud, if you like—then reflect on what they mean to you.

Bring your attention to the breath. Remember that at this time all you are is a breathing human being. Be aware of the oils, enjoy the scent, and feel how they affect your mind, body, emotions, and spirit.

When distractions arise, bring your attention gently back to your breathing. Don't try to suppress the thoughts and feelings that arise; simply be aware of them—don't indulge them, just let them flow by.

In your "disciplined silence" what does your inner wisdom tell you?

If you feel bliss or ecstatic joy inspired by Rumi's words, the vaporized oils, and your meditation, then enjoy the sensation. However, be aware these pleasant feelings will pass, and remain mindful of your breath.

Don't worry if you feel uninspired, puzzled, or simply quiet. We cannot conjure up spiritual feelings on demand; whatever you feel is right here and now for you.

When you are ready to finish, spend a few moments simply being and breathing.

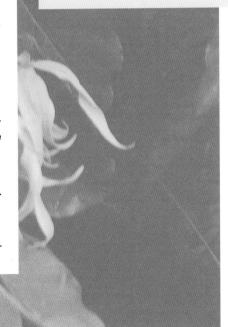

*"Not Christian or Jew or Muslim,
    not Hindu,
        Buddhist, sufi or zen.
Not any religion or cultural
        system...
I do not exist, am not an entity in
        this world or the next...
I belong to the beloved, have
        seen the two worlds as one
        and that one call to and know,
        first last, outer inner, only that
        breath breathing human being."*

**RUMI: "ONLY BREATH"
(EXCERPTS)**

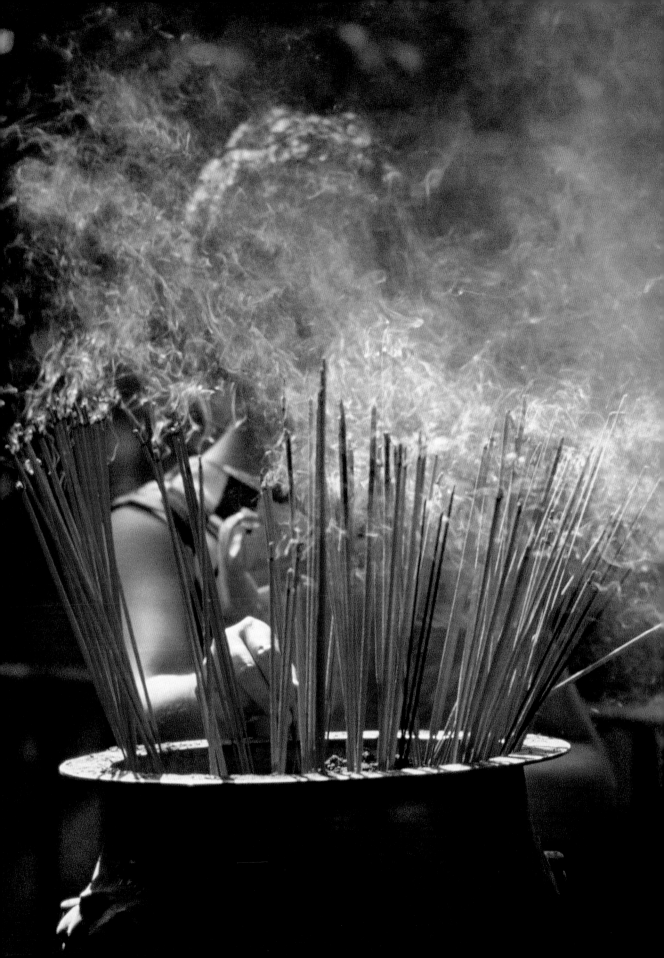

Ritual: Perfumes for the Gods

With today's global communications we have access to more knowledge than ever before, including the rituals, religions, and customs of every culture, both ancient and contemporary. This is a fascinating and unprecedented opportunity to draw from this priceless resource whatever rituals we can make meaningful in our lives. Rituals transform myths into a living dynamic reality, and when we hit on a ritual that is right for us we will recognize it, because archetypal images and nuggets of universal truth will flood from our unconscious mind into our waking consciousness, affecting spiritual renewal.

mythic

"If we strip off the tired and repetitive robot-like rituals that surround us, we have the priceless legacy of a varied and infinite store of knowledge, mythologies, patterns, **images**, and ideas from which to pick and choose in creating our own individual and highly charged mythic/ritual system."

DENNY SARGENT: *GLOBAL RITUALISM*

What is Ritual?

"Rituals are, and always have been, an important part of all cultures. Ancient cultures used herbs and aromatic plants for cooking, cleaning, health, to ward off evil spirits, as well as sacred ceremonies and to embalm the dead and see them off on their spirit journey to the next world."

JANINE MURPHY:
AROMATHERAPY TODAY, VOL 7

RITUALS ARE ACTIONS PERFORMED REGULARLY with conscious and unconscious expectations. They may have religious significance, in which case they probably follow an established ceremony in a long-standing tradition. Our conscious expectations of going to church include fulfilling the need to worship, satisfying the demands of family or culture, and receiving blessings. Such rituals also give us a forum to communicate with the gods and to consider the meaning of life and death, even though our ponderings often remain unconscious.

However, many rituals are part of daily life. This does not mean they are less spiritually powerful, unless we remain blind to their potential. All rituals focus and activate our inner power. Ritual

characteristics include cycles of repetitive actions performed in a specific way that do not have strong functional or logical content, but do have strong personal meaning. In this way rituals allow us to act out our personal myths and inner dramas, creating a dynamic reality with individual significance.

Primitive cultures used ritual as a means of creating reality. The ancient caveman hunter was aware of the dangers of hunting the wild animals that provided his food and clothing. Not only might he get hurt in the fight, but he had to find tracks and perhaps spend many days in pursuit. The longer the chase, the more hungry he became. Successful hunting meant survival; failure meant death. So the caveman prepared himself psychologically, using ritual magic to help him achieve his goal.

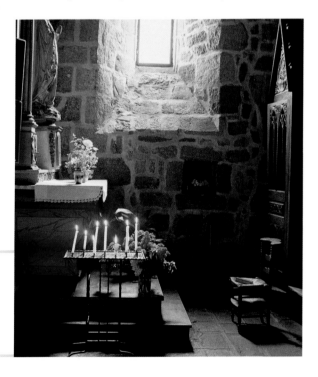

Attending church

When we attend a church service we fulfill our conscious expectations of worship and receiving God's blessing, as well as satisfying the demands of family and culture.

Cave painting

The ancient cave painting of hands at Cuevos Los Manos, Argentina, was part of our ancestor's rituals to create spiritual meaning, as well as a form of artistic expression.

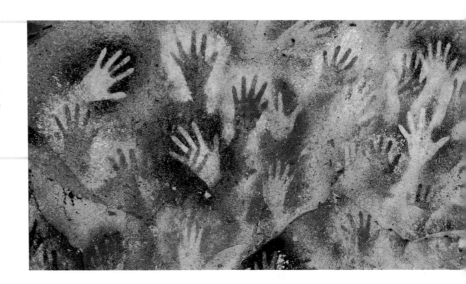

Ritual significance of cave art

The cave paintings we admire today were more than decoration. They were ritually painted images summoned up from the collective psyche and the painter's imagination and memory. The painting was accompanied by ritual prayers for the animals to appear; literally, the appearance of the animal on the cave wall was a psychic summoning of a real animal. When the painting was finished, anthropologists assume that the hunter would ritually stab it, symbolizing a successful hunt; they also think that when he hunted he may have believed the power of his rituals would bring the reality of the animal he had imaginatively created.

We still create our own reality to some extent. For example, if the violinist who ritually practices for a concert doesn't make herself believe she can perform her piece perfectly, she knows she will falter. Training for a virtuoso performance has a ritual element, which includes psychological programming to stimulate the artist's confidence in his or her ability to give a perfect performance.

However, this is not the only purpose of secular ritual. We are all familiar with our family or group rituals, including shared meals and birthday parties, in which we are united in celebrating life together. Equally important is the power of ritual to bring about change; the process of ritual can lead us to see that our original goal is not always so important. Thus, as much as affirming belief systems, ritual can affect personal and social development.

Making changes can be hard, and those that instigate change—rather than those who impose it like dictators—often exist on the fringes of society: the visionaries, artists, shamans, mystics, and free spirits whose gifted visions are usually appreciated only long after they are dead. Through their often tortured spiritual journeys the finest of these personal ritual expressions become accepted into mainstream society, breathing new life into our culture.

Different Ritual Traditions

*"I mean, try to explain to someone
why we have this odd cultural
tradition of smoking after dinner, or
why we knock on wood for luck."*

DENNY SARGENT: *GLOBAL RITUALISM*

THE HISTORY OF RITUAL IS WIDESPREAD THROUGH
the great religions of the world, and in many small
esoteric tribal groups. The most prevalent Christian
ritual is participation in the Eucharist, where the
congregation believes that Christ's body becomes
present in the sacramental bread and his blood in the
sacramental wine. In Tibetan Buddhist Lama Dances
a similar transformation takes place, with spirits
entering ritual implements and being subdued.

Aromatics are often burned during religious
rituals—such as the burning of frankincense during
Catholic services and incense in Hindu and Buddhist
rituals. Another form of aromatic ritual is practiced by
several African tribes, who anoint their bodies with
scented oil, combining moisturizing sun protection
and perfuming alongside pleasing their gods.

The most sophisticated religious ritual using
aromatics was ancient Egyptian embalming. This
combined a belief in immortality, which subscribed to
the assumption that the deceased journeyed to
another existence, together with the desire to keep the
body as much like it was in life as possible. This
sophisticated and expensive process was reserved for
royalty and high priests. It spawned an entire
industry, the knowledge and rituals of which
overlapped with the cosmetic and perfume industries.

Some rituals incorporate strong hygienic and
health considerations. In countries with cooler
climates religious funerals include burial, but in
hotter climates cremation is usual. In Tibet's cold,
harsh climate, Tibetan Buddhist "sky burial" was
normal. This involved chopping up the body to feed
to the birds—a last act of generosity that would lead
to a positive rebirth. After the Chinese invasion of
Tibet, many Tibetans fled to India where the climate
is unsuitable for disposal of corpses by this method.
Now the custom is ritual cremation, similar to the
traditional Indian system. Religious ritual can adapt
according to changing circumstances.

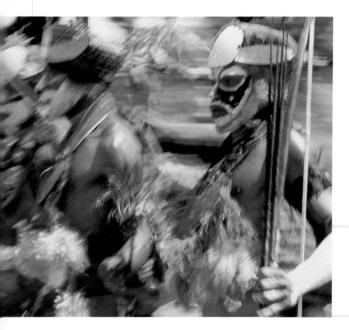

Tribal ceremony

This colorful ritual at Mount Hagen Sing-sing, Papua New
Guinea, is full of ritual significance to the participants.

Superstition and ritual

In a modern world based on logic and empirical reasoning, many of us have driven our superstitious rituals into our unconscious, yet we almost all fall prey to one every once in a while. When you spill salt do you perhaps throw a pinch over your left shoulder? If so, are you aware that this ritual derives from a belief that God stands behind your right shoulder and Satan behind your left?

Another superstition is that breaking a mirror gives you seven years of bad luck—which rested on the belief that your reflected image had some reality in the first place. It was commonly believed that it took the body seven years to regenerate all its cells and that seven was a magical number. But if you break a mirror today, this old superstition often still springs to mind. Our cultural rituals are strongly embedded in our unconscious and our collective psyche—whether we like it or not!

We all have our personal daily rituals that we have made part of our lives, and we tend to get upset when we are forced to break our ritual habits such as missing a customary early morning cup of tea. If a man's daily newspaper is sold out at his local newsdealer, he may get annoyed; even though there are other newspapers that will give him roughly the same news, "his" paper is gone—along with his ritual.

Rituals can be of much benefit to us, once we accept their influence and perform them consciously with the proper intention, and in the correct way. Rituals are part of being human, and whether these are group or personal rituals, the rituals with essential oils described in this chapter can empower us and enhance our lives.

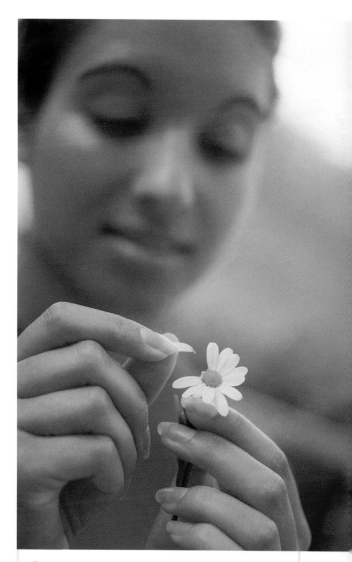

Superstition

This woman is playing the traditional superstitious game of "He loves me, he loves me not." She will recite the two phrases alternately as she pulls off each petal; the phrase she uses when she pulls off the final petal, according to superstition, reveals the feelings of the man in question.

Why Ritual is Useful Today

"The Chewong Shaman takes some of the incense smoke in his fist, puts his fist to his mouth and blows in four directions, after which he prays to the spirits for divine protection. The smoke is believed to carry the shaman's words up to the spirit world."

C. CLASSEN: *AROMATHERAPY TODAY, VOL 13*

THOUGH WE MIGHT THINK OF SPIRITUAL RITUALS IN the past tense, this is a modern Western fallacy. Many cultures have daily rituals that are part of normal life to them and seem strange only to us. I imagine our computer and television "rituals" seem equally strange to them! For example, the Chewongs of the Malay Peninsula attract and "feed" good spirits with an offering of burnt fragrant wood every night.

Some of our everyday actions are rituals, or at least can be when we do them with conscious intent. Things we do every day that we take for granted can become substantially enriched experiences by taking a little time to think about what it is we are doing, why and how we are doing it, and what our expectations are. Ritual is about transforming the mundane.

Let's look at the shower many of us take every morning. Often we stumble out of bed into the shower, wait impatiently for the water to reach the right temperature, and then wash perfunctorily. We are not aware of what we are doing; perhaps we do not even enjoy it. Yet the morning shower can be a nurturing ritual, preparing mind, body, and spirit for the day ahead.

Another way to shower is to regard it as a morning ritual, washing away the detritus of sleep and awakening to the new day. Sprinkle six to eight drops of essential oil on the shower floor just before you get in and the fragrance will mingle with the steam that envelops you. Choose your oils carefully to reflect how you feel and to prepare you for the day ahead. Sprinkle them mindfully, shower with awareness, feel the sensation of the water and the oils, and embrace the experience. Quite a difference!

Take time to enjoy the sensation. Mindfully consider each part of your body, find areas of tension, and relax them. Breathe in the vaporized oils and visualize them entering your body through your skin and lungs, bringing healing relaxation.

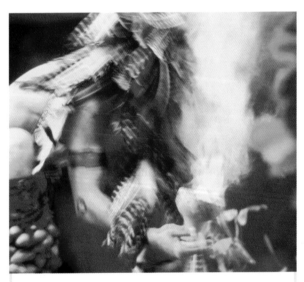

Shaman

This Mayan shaman is performing a sacred ritual in Xcaret Eco Park. His deep concentration and conscious awareness of his actions contribute greatly to his ritual.

Cleansing

We can treat our daily shower as a cleansing ritual, and enjoy it a lot more, using essential oils to enhance the experience.

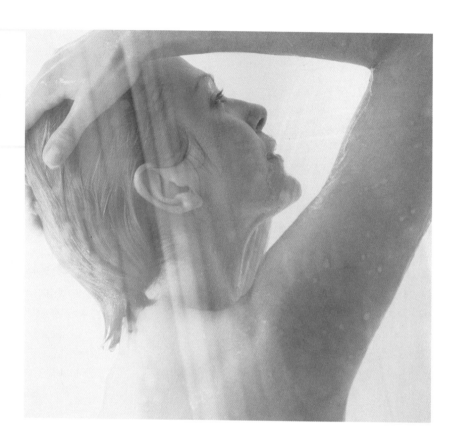

Bringing ritual into consciousness

Ritual and meditation have several common features, the most important of which is they help us to live our lives consciously in the present. Meditation is a part of all rituals, and many meditations can have a ritual aspect. Through meditation and ritual we can discover our own spiritual side, our own gods or higher wisdom, and honor these in our daily lives.

Bringing ritual into our hectic modern lifestyle helps us to enjoy what we often dismiss as boring, practical tasks. By taking time to see them in another way, and really being present while doing them, grounds us in what it means to be alive. For example, if we think of washing the dishes after dinner, we usually don't feel like doing it. However, if we choose to wash dishes as part of a ritual meal, and can understand the significance of it, then we can transform the act.

What we normally rush through wishing we were elsewhere can become a new experience, as we mindfully and ritually clean up. This rediscovering of our life beyond the daily rushing to work, the crashing out in front of the television, the escapism through alcohol, can bring lasting inner peace and happiness.

Preparation, Banishing, and Purification

"We must stress the fact that scents do not put the individual into a state of trance. In the judicious choice of aromatics, there is no danger of abuse. It is no less true to say that the use of perfumes sharpens the perception sometimes beyond the ordinary."

MARGUERITE MAURY: *MARGUERITE MAURY'S GUIDE TO AROMATHERAPY*

ALL RITUALS REQUIRE PROPER PREPARATION; rushing into something potentially powerful before you are ready is foolish. Preparation in this sense is inner preparation; we will look at outer preparation in Creating a Sacred Space (see pages 106–107). Inner preparation is meditation, and this centers and grounds your energies, and strengthens your focus. This is accomplished by a period of mindful awareness meditation.

Once your mind is calm and clear, turn your attention to what you hope to achieve through your ritual, what the intentions and objectives are. This is a creative process—you may not have clear intent at this stage. Your vision of the ritual becomes clear as you draw on inner wisdom and inspiration from higher forces. Your unconscious desires have the space to come through into consciousness, and unite with the conscious will to accomplish the ritual successfully.

This is called psychic centering in some traditions, and draws together the intention, objective, vision, will, and belief in the ritual. In many ways this process is the most important part of the ritual, and without it the ritual may not succeed. This inner envisioning of the ritual ensures that what you want to achieve is realistic, and gives space to modify any aspect of the ritual until you know intuitively that everything is right and you are ready to begin.

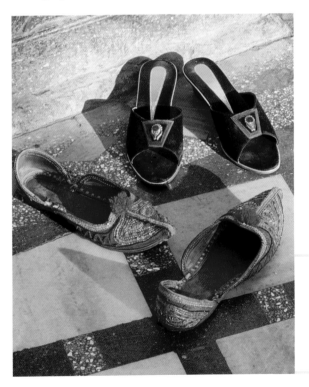

Shoe symbolism

It is customary to remove your shoes when entering a temple or shrine in the East. Not only does this leave the physical dirt outside, it symbolizes leaving behind concerns from the outside world.

Banishing

Banishing is the elimination of unwanted thoughts, energies, spirits, spiritual pollution, and bad luck. Some rituals require a lengthy, complex banishing, or purification, but the simple rituals dealt with here need only basic purification. The purpose of banishing is to purify the person spiritually before she or he enters the sacred space in which the ritual will take place. This means clearing both the conscious and unconscious mind of distractions, insecurities, and worries before the ritual commences. In some cultures this is described as banishing evil spirits, or driving out demons, and it can be useful to regard obsessive thoughts in this way.

In this way banishing reinforces the clear, focused concentration developed from the mindful awareness meditation. This is the inner psychological aspect of banishing that is then strengthened by an outer physical act. The physical aspect of banishing needs to be symbolic of the inner purification in order to be effective.

This is simple to achieve. For example, before entering Eastern temples, whether they are Shinto, Hindu, Muslim, or Buddhist, you remove your shoes, which symbolizes leaving behind not only the physical dirt from outside but also mental "dirt," i.e. concerns from the outside world. Some sacred places require that your head is covered or bowed as a sign of respect. Shinto shrines require that you rinse your mouth and wash your hands with water before entering; washing is a strong symbol of purification.

It is best to choose a personal banishing act with which you feel comfortable and which symbolizes purification for you. The simple act of washing the hands with running water may be sufficient. You can also rinse your mouth with water—a strong symbolic act of purifying speech. If the ritual is inside, then removing your shoes makes good sense. You can devise your own personal banishing, too; what is important is that it works for you.

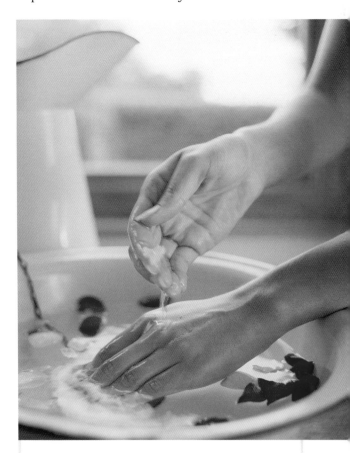

Washing hands

The simple act of washing the hands can be an effective banishing or purification if it is performed consciously with the intent of purification.

Rituals with Essential Oils

"Almost all human cultures have used and continue to use incense in numerous social situations and religious or spiritual rituals... Sacred rites of smell are common to many peoples. In Mexico, the Tzotzil people dedicate to their deities candles and copal incense."

SALVATORE BATTAGLIA:
AROMATHERAPY TODAY, VOL 13

RITUALS USING ESSENTIAL OILS FOLLOW THE tradition of sacred rituals from antiquity to the present day. Offering essential oils instead of incense on your altar allows you to use the qualities of the oils to influence your mood, assist your meditation, and alleviate stress and anxiety. However, you are also offering them to your gods—whoever or whatever they may be—and the act of preparing the burner with the candle and the oils should be done ritually and in honor of God, Buddha, Isis, or another higher being.

Ritual bathing with essential oils is not a new invention, but a timely revival to counteract the stresses of modern living. A ritual bath involves a lot more than simply running the bath, throwing in a random selection of oils, and leaping in and out in five minutes! The preparation is itself a ritual that readies you to appreciate the ritual bathing experience fully.

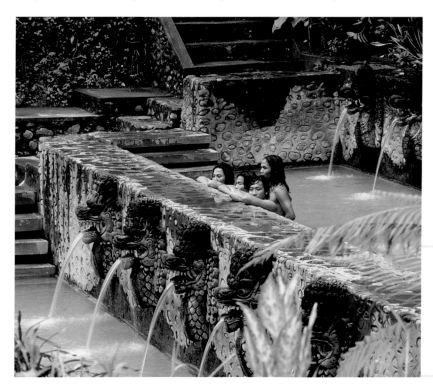

Hot springs

Rituals involving water represent purification and are widespread throughout the world. Here, a group of people relax in a hot spring in Bali, Indonesia.

Ritual bathing with essential oils

Take a quick shower first, and wash with soap. A ritual bath with essential oils is more relaxing and effective if cleansing is done beforehand; this follows the custom of group bathing practiced in Japan, and hot tubs in California. The shower is also an appropriate banishing before the bath ritual.

Now you are ready to transform your bathroom into a sacred space. Any ritual using water involves purification, so we add other objects to reinforce the purifying effect. Lit candles are renowned for cleansing the aura, and their gentle light is preferable to electric. Place candles mindfully around the room, including the edge of the bath if it is wide enough to hold them safely. Light as many as you wish.

Other natural objects are also suitable, particularly crystals that reflect the flickering life of the candles. Beautiful stones are effective and provide a grounding influence. Plants and flowers echo the origins of the essential oils and keep the atmosphere vibrant. Let your imagination run riot; your intuition will help your conscious ideas about where to place your ritual ornaments.

As you prepare your space, let your mind wander into the realm of essential oils and discover which you want to use. If nothing clear comes through, meditate for a few minutes while the water is running. When you turn on the faucets, be mindful of how precious water is, how lucky you are to be

"Here first she bathes, and round her body pours Soft oils of fragrance and ambrosial showers..."

HOMER

able to simply turn a faucet when many others must work to get their water.

When your space is prepared and your bath is run it is time to put in the oils. Six to eight drops is sufficient, four to six if you are including spice oils or absolutes. Mix them into a small amount of base bath oil, or drop them directly in the water. Agitate the water to disperse the oils, remembering that they don't dissolve in water and be careful not to get neat oil on your skin. Slowly immerse yourself in the water, and enjoy your ritual bath.

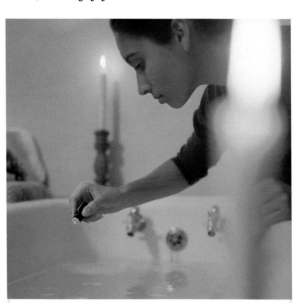

Ritual bath
Bathing with essential oils is very calming. The preparations beforehand are integral to the ritual.

Developing Inner Wisdom through Ritual Play

"Each essence has its own personality, its own set of attributes, and this can be used to bring out certain qualities in us; helping us to see ourselves more clearly, to understand our faults, and to let the beauty and joy of our souls breathe a fresh, summery fragrance through our minds."

ROBERT TISSERAND:
THE ART OF AROMATHERAPY

ESSENTIAL OILS ARE THE SOULS OF PLANTS, and we should remain conscious of this. In ancient civilizations healing was considered a sacred art practiced as a ritual by priests or priestesses using aromatic plants ascribed to the Divine. Essential oils are living organic substances, and they subtly respond according to how they are treated; if their sacred nature is honored, they stay vibrant and powerful.

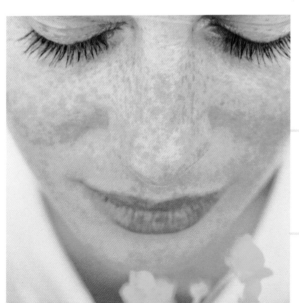

If you use an essential oil continuously its power will dwindle, but this will return if you take a break. This makes it important to keep a range of oils, try out different blends, and simply play with them. Too often we impose limits on ourselves, and rediscovering the child within is liberating. Our inner child helps us find our inner wisdom through a willingness to play and explore.

Often we don't know where to start, so it may help to return to the magical realm of child play. I remember buying my first essential oils and unconsciously sitting on the floor to explore the individually wrapped little bottles. As I unwrapped them the sun's rays caught the glass and threw light across the room. As I opened each bottle carefully and smelled the essential oil inside I was enthralled— just like a child.

We can find a balance between reverence and fun in experimenting with essential oils. If we are not careful, their highly concentrated power can hurt us, but if we are too controlled we will never learn how to unlock their secrets. Sacred ritual is about going beyond the individual "I" or ego, and connecting with the higher self or collective unconscious, intuition, and higher wisdom. Sacrificing our personal ego during ritual is a small price to pay to open up to the universal energies around us.

Inner child
The combination of meditation and innocent appreciation of nature helps us connect with our inner child. The open-mindedness of the child helps us discover our latent wisdom.

Choosing oils

Learning about the different essential oils through ritual play helps us when we need to select individual oils for our meditations and rituals.

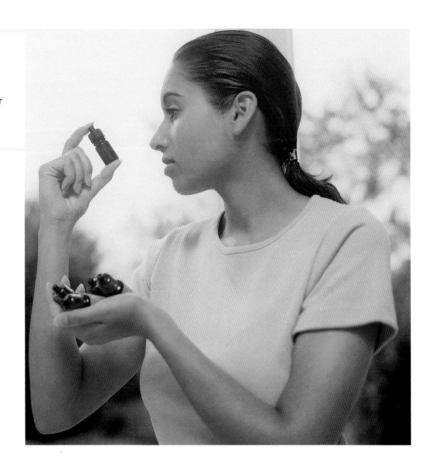

Ritual as sacred play

Try playing with your oils sitting on the floor. Watch how your adult mind wants to label and judge—for example: "this is an absolute." Try to let go of this. Enjoy the sunlight reflecting off the colored glass. Pick a bottle at random and open it without looking at the label. Smell the oil and guess what it is. Write down words and images that spring to mind—summer breeze, forests, vacations in France.

When you look to see what it is, keep your associations. They will help you far more than the name when it comes to choosing oils for meditations and rituals. Pour a drop onto a cotton ball. What color is this essential oil? Is it thin like water or thick and slow to pour? Does this tell you anything about the nature of the essential oil? Do you feel an affinity with it?

Play with only a few oils at a time because our sense of smell wears out quickly, but play as often as you like. You could read the descriptions of the oils with your associations. But most important, you are developing your intuition, your inner wisdom, and this will help you to choose the oils that are right for you for each meditation and ritual.

Creating a Sacred Space

*"A danger with ritual is that
instead of contributing to a sense
of awakening and presence, it can
have a numbing effect. Yet
engagement in rituals can open
up our consciousness. It might be
that we resist religious ritual
without ever taking the time to
experience it."*

CHRISTOPHER TITMUSS:
THE POWER OF MEDITATION

AFTER BANISHING, THE INNER PURIFICATION, IT IS time to create the sacred space, a means of achieving outer purification. Ritual works by being on another plane, away from the clutter of daily life, free from mundane reality. This reflects the creation of sacred space in your mind accomplished by meditation, and the two spaces resonate harmoniously.

Sacred space is often described as a place between the worlds where the divine and the earthly can meet. Privacy is important, so the place and time chosen for your ritual need careful thought. The space is not necessarily intrinsically sacred, but your preparations make it so. Clearing away all your ritual objects at the end brings the space back to normality. This is important if you are ritually bathing in a shared bathroom, for example; the energies from the ritual must be freed so that the place is psychically clean for the next person.

Your altar is a sacred place, too. Strong, peaceful energies may develop around it and create an atmosphere similar to that which we find in a church or temple. If the ritual is outside, you may find yourself intuitively drawn to a spot that may have once been used for ritual or religious services, or it may simply be a place where Nature's powers have congregated. These natural sacred places are ideal for ritual, and you may wish to return to them time and again.

Almost any physical space can be sacred depending on our inner mental, emotional, and psychic space. By directing our perception inward through meditation, centering and focusing our energies, we contribute to making the outer environment sacred. Our intention for the ritual, along with our concentration, can make a natural beauty spot or an ordinary room as sacred as a temple.

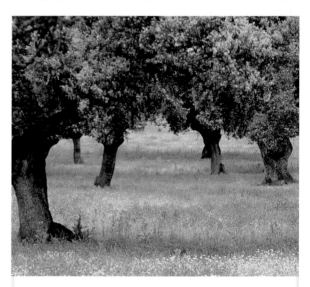

Beauty spot
Natural sacred places, such as this beautiful grove of trees, are ideal for ritual. You may feel intuitively drawn to such a place, where Nature's energies tend to congregate.

Purifying and defining sacred spaces

Preparation is an important part of the ritual and should not be rushed. The first step is cleaning and purifying, the second is delineating and marking the boundaries. After these are accomplished, you bring in essential oils and other objects you may want to use such as crystals, vessels of water, and candles. If you are outside, you may like to light a fire, if this is fitting.

Cleansing the sacred space involves both physical cleaning and purifying psychic energy. If the ritual is inside, clean the floor and all surfaces. If it is outside, brush away dead leaves, twigs, and dirt. A good way to purify the air and psychic energy is to spray water around. If the sacred space feels contaminated—by the recent presence of another person or because it is simply dirty—then include some purifying essential oils, such as juniper or lemon, in the water.

In some magical rituals the drawing of particular shapes on the floor is necessary. However, for the simple rituals with essential oils described here, marking your boundaries is what is important. A sacred space cannot function as such if you are not clear where it starts and finishes. After a space is cleaned and prepared for indoor rituals, for example, shut the door mindfully. As you do so, be aware that all areas inside the room belong to the sacred space, everything outside the room does not.

If your ritual is outside, first meditate in the center of the space you have selected. Feel the energy, and visualize where the space starts and ends. When you are clear about the shape, size, and boundaries, the perimeter is then marked. If the shape is vague, use a circle; this is the most frequent shape for enclosing a ritual space. You can mark the boundaries with leaves, petals, salt, cornmeal, or something similar. Alternatively, water with or without essential oils can be dripped as you walk around mindfully creating your sacred space.

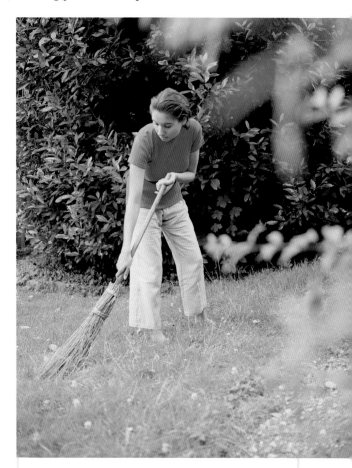

Clearing a space

When you are clearing a space outside, it is important to brush away dead leaves, twigs, and dirt. These preliminaries are an integral part of the ritual and should be done with mindful awareness.

Psychic Detoxification Bath Ritual

"Aromatic baths may affect us in a variety of ways. Firstly there is the fragrance of the essences used; if this is pleasing to the nose it will also please the spirit."

ROBERT TISSERAND:
THE ART OF AROMATHERAPY

IN THIS BATHING RITUAL YOU ARE WASHING away tiredness, stress, and perhaps, for example, psychic contamination from traveling home in a crowded train. Maybe your work involves contact with a lot of people, and this can be psychically wearing. This bath ritual is invaluable if you had an argument, or someone shouted at you, or was unpleasant to you during the day.

If you are tired and stressed, you should keep your preparations and choice of oils quick and simple; anything too elaborate at this stage may simply aggravate your stress level. If any essential oil or blend springs to mind, it is likely to be appropriate; a quick smell test will check this. Otherwise think of what you need and would like from your ritual aromatic bath. Take into account what you will be doing afterward—if you have to go out to dinner, for example, avoid oils that you know will make you sleepy.

Juniper is an obvious choice for detoxifying. If you don't want to use it in the bath, a simple banishing using juniper is a good alternative. Rub two or three drops of juniper between your palms and brush down your body while still clothed, starting at the head and covering all parts. This can be done either aurically—brushing the natural energy field close to your body—or touching your body, because the oils don't stain your clothes. Lemon, angelica, cedarwood, and rosewood can also be used for banishing in this way.

If you are tired, you will be sensitive, so include a delicate oil in your blend. Lavender combines light, refreshing qualities with deep relaxation; bergamot will lift your spirits. Neroli, rose, and melissa will soothe emotional pain if someone has been unpleasant to you; jasmine will restore your confidence if someone has been critical of your work. If you feel you might have trouble sleeping, chamomile, clary sage, marjoram, or narcissus will help. Frankincense, sandalwood, and mandarin slow racing thoughts.

Melissa

Melissa essential oil is useful in a psychic detoxification bath ritual, particularly if someone has recently been unpleasant to you. Melissa soothes emotional pain, reduces shock, and is sedative, calming, and antidepressant.

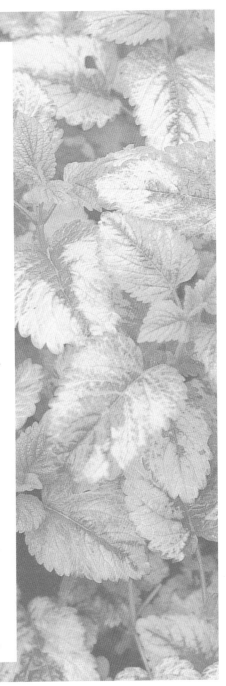

Aromatic Bath Ritual

Do a simple banishing or take a quick shower.

Start to run the water for your bath. Light candles and place them around the bathroom. Turn off electric lights.

Place at least one beautiful object where you can see it from the bath, such as a vase of flowers, a large crystal, or an image that holds spiritual meaning for you.

You might like to play some relaxing music quietly. Be careful not to choose music that will distract you, and keep the volume low. Gregorian chants, other spiritual, classical, or new age music are all suitable according to your preference.

When the bath is full, add your oils and agitate the water to disperse them.

Climb in mindfully. Feel the water swirl around your body, easing aches and stress.

Cup your hands—or use a bowl or pitcher—and pour water over your head repeatedly. This washes away psychic contamination and helps to purify the aura, so do this slowly and mindfully.

Lie back and enjoy the fragrance of the oils. Breathe deeply, and bring your attention to your breath. Let all your thoughts arise and pass, focus on your breathing and your body for as long as you wish.

Centering Energies

"Take a stick. Stand on a beach.
Clear your mind. Draw a circle.
It is the universe. Draw a cross in it.
You are HERE..."

DENNY SARGENT: *GLOBAL RITUALISM*

ALL RITUALS REQUIRE FOCUS, CONCENTRATION, AND inner centering of your energies. Many rituals also benefit from centering the physical sacred space. After marking the boundaries of your sacred space—especially for rituals outside—you can mark the four directions. This can be simple—a small pile of stones perhaps—or, if you have the inclination, it can be more complex. Keep in mind why you are doing it. This gives the center definition, which is important as a central focus of energies, and is the place you will start and end the ritual.

We can see from the sacred temples and places of worship from many different cultures how the four directions and the powers they embody are important. Sometimes these are visualized during the ritual, and offerings are made to invisible directional power spots. Native American rituals use the sacred pipe filled with tobacco, and, before this is ritually smoked and passed from participant to participant, it is offered to the four directions.

Sometimes the four directions are embodied in the place of worship; for example, Buddhist temples have four corner towers. Sometimes it is in the symbol itself, the most obvious being the cross. We think of this as Christian, but many tribal religions also used this symbol, and crossroads have always been held as places of power where energies from different directions meet, and where you can literally change direction.

The four directions are often symbolic of the elements, or represent protector deities who safeguard the sacred space from unwelcome energies or invaders. Sometimes rituals build on this system and have six directions (including up and down) or the interdirections are included, to make eight, or ten. They all define and protect the center, which is also symbolic of the person performing the ritual.

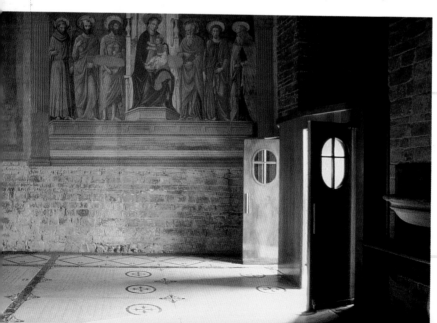

Sacred space

All temples and churches have respect for the four directions and the powers they embody, as shown in the symbol of the cross, for example. We can see this symbol here in the door windows of the San Miniato church in Florence, Italy.

Inner centering

Before you start the ritual you must have clear intent, followed by banishing. The first thing to do is to center your own energies through mindful awareness meditation. You can use essential oils to calm the mind and aid clarity and concentration. Appropriate oils are frankincense, lavender, patchouli, lemon, and holy basil.

Once your mind is calm, continue meditating to find, clarify and strengthen your intent. You can then do a banishing and create your sacred space. Before leaping into the ritual, go to the center of your sacred space. Acknowledge the four directions; this can be a simple bowing in each direction, or you might like to make an offering in the four directions. This defines the center within its own universe, so it is both spacious and contained. This helps you open to the energy of the sacred space, as well as to your own unconscious and intuition.

Spend some more time in mindfulness meditation to ground your energy and clear your mind, so that when you start the ritual you can give it your full attention. This helps you to find and develop your own inner power; the combination of clear intent and focused concentration within the sacred space is itself a "place of power." If you find this process daunting, first try the circle on the beach—or other open space—exercise in the quotation (*see* top left).

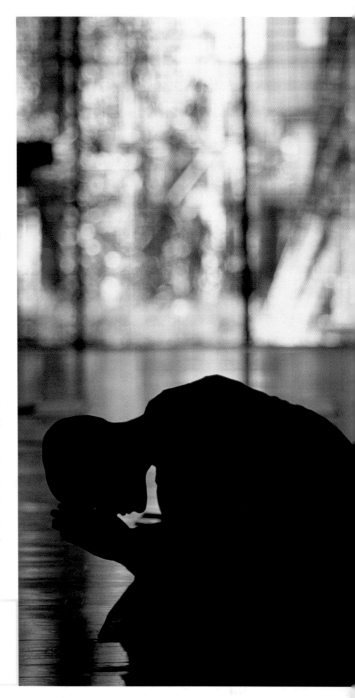

Inner space
We create our own inner space, where we center our energies, through meditation.

Ritual Intimate Massage for Lovers

"With aromantic massage, a sexual feeling, spontaneity and instinct are worth infinitely more than a degree course in massage technique."

VALERIE ANN WORWOOD: *AROMANTICS*

TOUCH IS A VITAL PART OF COMMUNICATION between lovers; a squeezed hand can say more than a hundred words. Massage is healing and nurturing, but can also be stimulating and erotic. Intention plays an important role in all rituals. Sometimes sexual feelings require urgent expression; at other times, they require slow, erotic foreplay. Ritual intimate massage—and the preparations—falls into the latter category, though you do not have to make love afterward; this is a choice for both people.

If you are unfamiliar with aromatherapy massage, these guidelines will help ensure your massage is uninterrupted pleasure. You must have intent, purification, a sacred place, and centered energies. Ensure the proposed time and place suit both people; if one is too tired, the experience will be limited.

Both people should bathe or shower first for banishing. Do this alone; it will increase anticipation. Your sacred space might be your bedroom, or perhaps living room if you have a working fireplace. In either case, make sure the room

is clean, and very warm—oiled naked flesh chills surprisingly quickly, even in the heat of passion. Candles, beautiful objects, and low music all help to create a suitable atmosphere.

Prepare your massage blend shortly beforehand. In a small dish mix 0.7 fl oz (20 ml) of almond oil with up to twelve drops of essential oil. You will probably know by now which oils you find erotic, but here are few blends you might like to try: neroli, clary sage, and bergamot; jasmine, sandalwood, and mandarin; ylang ylang, rosewood, and ginger; linden blossom, lemon, and frankincense; violet leaf, rose, and sandalwood.

If you will be massaging on the floor, fold a quilt and cover it with towels. If you use the bed, cover sheets, quilts, and pillows with towels. Have other towels at hand to cover the parts of the body not being massaged. Wear loose clothes or no clothes. Turn off the phone and you are ready to begin.

Intimate massage

Ritual massage between lovers can be as erotic as you like, or it can be simply loving, caring, and nurturing, creating a safe haven from the outside world.

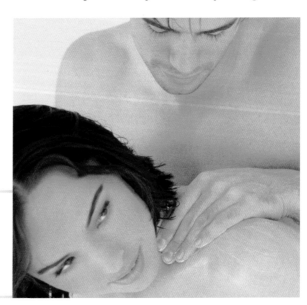

Intimate Massage Ritual

When you are both ready and the room is prepared, spend a few minutes in mindful meditation together to center your energies and clear your mind. This also gives you time to reflect on your love for each other.

Uncover your partner's back slowly. To start the massage, dip your hands in the oil; never pour oil directly onto someone—it feels horrible.

Kneel comfortably to one side, or sit on your partner's buttocks if he or she can bear your weight easily. Starting at the base, use both hands to do long, smooth strokes up the back then down in a rhythmic flow.

Slow, firm, continuous strokes feel best. Ask your partner how he or she feels, and adjust pressure accordingly.

When you feel ready to move on, cover the back, and ask which part your partner would like massaged next, or whether it is time to swap over.

Be mindful of giving and receiving loving massage. Allow sexual excitement to exist and grow, you don't have to rush in immediately.

Delight in the erotic perfume of the oils and the sensation of the massage. If and when you both feel ready to make love, make sure the bowl of oil is somewhere close, where you can smell the oils, but not where you will knock it over.

Invocation, Evocation, or Magic

"Always remember essential oils are highly volatile, very powerful natural essences. They have very high vibrational energy. Working with them is like working with magic. And what is magic? Magic is energy."

JANINE MURPHY:
AROMATHERAPY TODAY, VOL 7

INVOCATION, EVOCATION, OR MAGIC ARE AT the center of every ritual, however simple. In practice, many rituals involve two or all three of these in various combinations. Although these exotic-sounding words conjure up a fantastic scene of magicians in robes wrestling with demons, this scene is only fantasy or belongs to advanced ritualists. The simple rituals with essential oils shown here work with the souls of plants and their inherent powers, in a far less dramatic manner.

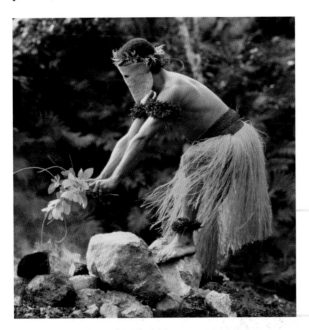

Invocation is when we behave in such a way as to summon to our level a cosmic force, god, goddess, or superior being that belongs to a plane of existence higher than our own. This being or spirit comes from outside the person, attracted by the power of the ritual. An example of invocation is spirit possession of the hougan, or priest, during a voodoo ritual. During possession it is the spirit that manifests; the priest is temporarily submerged by the higher power.

Evocation is when our ritual summons a cosmic force, an archetypal god/goddess figure, or spirit which manifests from inside our own continuum, and with which we then identify. This can be a being of a higher or lower order than ourselves. During the ritual we act as the spirit evoked; our own ego is temporarily on hold, though experienced ritualists can control some spirits. An example of evocation is the shaman who puts herself into a trance and then feels the presence of a Nature god arise within her.

How do invocation and evocation function in our simple rituals with essential oils? If our intent is to connect with the natural power of the oil, and we meditate on this, we energize our consciousness to be receptive to the soul of the plant. This is reinforced if we visualize what the plant looks like while burning the oil and so on. With practice, we learn to feel its presence in us, or in the surrounding atmosphere.

Invocation and evocation

This young Fijian witch doctor is making fire in a sacred outdoor setting in Viti Levu, Fiji. This is part of a complex ritual in which the witch doctor will contact his local spirits.

Magic with essential oils

Essential oils have an inherent magic, as the description "the souls of plants" implies. Rituals with oils strengthen this, if we think of magic as energy and the willed transformation of energy. Magic cannot be "black" or "white" by itself; the intention of the person performing the ritual classifies it.

Some aromatherapy books describe essential oils as magic potions. The essence of the plant is distilled from the plant mass into a tiny amount of essential oil, then secreted away into little bottles and tightly sealed with a dropper and cap. As we open a bottle of essential oil it starts to vaporize, like the genie wafting out of a bottle.

When we are using essential oils, if we are able to focus on their power, we should be able to bring into consciousness their magical qualities. Then, however we use them, their magic can help transform our energy and our consciousness—creating relaxation from stress, and calm concentration from a distracted mind.

The modern aromatherapist can be likened to a witch, because both follow the tradition of healing with plants. Using essential oils in ritual and meditation also forms part of the repertoire of those involved in witchcraft. Rituals with essential oils tap into this ancient tradition and increase our inner strength and creativity.

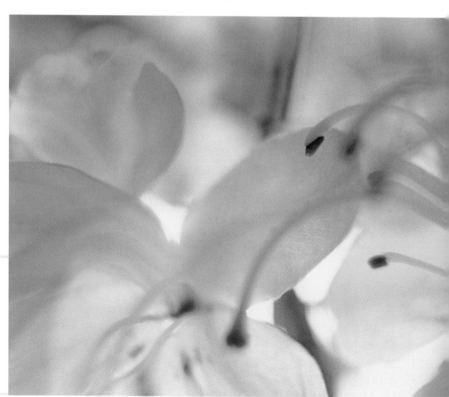

Magical flowers
Flowers appear every spring as part of the magic of Nature. Those that produce essential oils provide us with magic potions for healing, meditation, and ritual.

Seasonal and Psychic Cleaning Rituals

"...rituals should be joyful; don't make them into long-faced, over-solemn sessions. If anything goes wrong, simply start again, or backtrack a page and pick up the thread. If it's funny, laugh—you won't get struck down."

DOLORES ASHCROFT-NOWICKI:
FIRST STEPS IN RITUAL

SPRING CLEANING CAN BE EXTENDED TO INCLUDE all seasons, though the focus is on ritual cleaning not housework. The four seasons are demarcated by summer and winter solstices, and spring and fall equinoxes. These are traditionally powerful dates on which to perform rituals, especially those that honor the passing and arising of Nature's seasons, and this is the intent of these rituals.

Choose the room you wish to perform the ritual in. A ritual on midsummer's night would ideally be in a room facing the setting sun. Time is important, and on midsummer's night you can time the ritual to cover the threshold between light and dark.

Banishing requires you to clean the room, and, if done mindfully with a sense of the importance of the occasion, this is joyful and an important part of the ritual! All participants—one person or more—should

shower or bathe. Now prepare the room, making the space sacred, by making it welcoming and beautiful. Select spiritual objects, flowers, plants, crystals, and candles, and so on according to the season. At fall equinox, you could include leaves and berries.

Start with a few minutes of mindful meditation, then bring to mind the season that is passing. Reflect what this means in Nature, then for you personally. Turn your attention to the incoming season and reflect on the meaning of it. Feel a part of the flow and mystery of Nature.

Prepare the burner with a seasonal offering of essential oils. For spring use green herbs like basil or rosemary; use floral oils for summer; citrus fruits in the fall; and in the winter use spice oils. Offer the lit burner at the four corners. You can read poetry, or play music that evokes the season during the directional offering. Place the burner in the center of the room, and end the ritual with meditation.

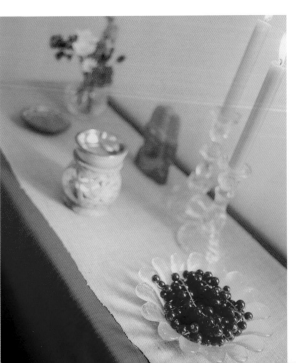

Summer altar
This summer altar encapsulates the spirit of the season with freshly picked red currants and a variety of summer flowers. You would burn summer floral essential oils in the burner.

Psychic room cleansing ritual

When you move into a new house, or room, the presence of the last occupant needs to be exorcised. This doesn't mean the previous person was evil, merely that you need clean space for the room to accept your energy and identity. We continually need to create our own sacred spaces that are free from mundane distractions and give us our "personal space." Some cultures describe the psychic cleansing of a room as driving out ghosts, and if you are sensitive to atmospheres you probably know what this means.

When you first enter the room, open the windows wide. Even in the winter, do this for five minutes. Clean the room, contemplating that this ritual is saying goodbye to the old presence and making space for your new presence. With the door and windows firmly shut, light a candle and mark the boundaries of your territory by holding the flame near the walls and slowly walking around the entire room.

Put out a few personal possessions you identify with strongly. Bring to mind essential oils and intuitively make a selection to cleanse the room psychically. Certain oils are indicated, such as juniper, lemon, geranium, cedarwood, and rosemary, but since this is your personal space the oils must reflect who you are.

Light the burner in the center of the room, and meditate beside it, feeling how the space has been cleansed of old energy. Visualize the oils vaporizing into the whole room. Become aware that the space is now your own sanctuary from the outside world. Animals mark their territory, and this ritual connects us with our natural instincts in a similar way.

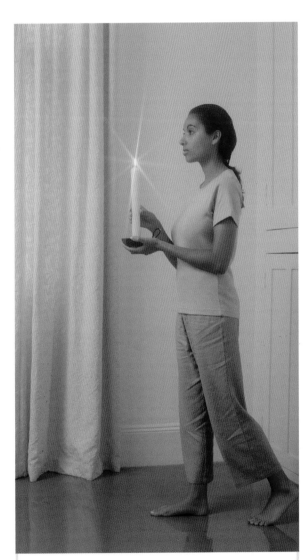

Marking boundaries

By holding a lighted candle close to the walls and walking carefully and slowly around the room we psychically make the room into our own personal space. Using a lighted candle—naked flame—is powerful; this makes us centered, focused, and careful.

Offerings and Endings

*"Simple gratitude for abundance,
as illustrated by... the Daiensai
or first rice offering in Japan,
or the Abundant Fruits
offering in Ancient China, always
seems to come from mankind
in a ritual way when the Earth gives
forth bounty."*

DENNY SARGENT: *GLOBAL RITUALISM*

WHEN YOU MEDITATE OR PERFORM A RITUAL with essential oils, there is always an element of offering the essential oils to Nature, a god, or higher wisdom being. Offerings are about the exchange of energy; you receive according to what and how you give. Energy is never wasted, it always goes somewhere as we know from Einstein's famous theory of relativity. But for an offering to be efficacious, the attitude and belief of the person making it is important too.

There is no point in offering inferior essential oils; in fact it is traditional to offer the best (or first) of whatever you are offering. There is also no point making the offering half-heartedly, or in a hurry, or because you think you ought to, rather than want to. If the attitude behind the offering is lacking, the ritual will also be lacking; in other words, you won't have fully achieved what you intended.

The offering of essential oils is also appreciated by the person making the offering, as you too enjoy the divine smells wafting up to the heavens. However, we can move away from the dualistic vision of superior god up there in heaven and inferior devotee down below. Whenever you make offerings you are also—and most importantly—acknowledging your own inner wisdom—the god within.

Ritual offerings bring the Divine without and the Divine within together. There is a saying in the Western esoteric tradition: "As above, so below," which encapsulates this. We make offerings consciously, and offer the finest essential oils to please and perfume the heaven above and the heaven below.

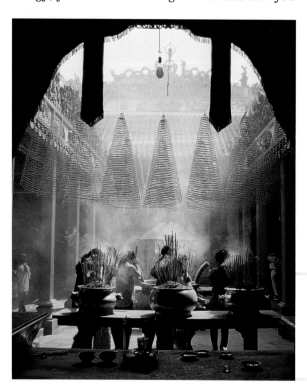

Offerings

Clouds of smoke from burnt offerings ascend to the god realms during this ritual at the Cholon Chinese Temple in Saigon, Vietnam.

Concluding rituals

The Greek philospher Aristotle said that every good story has a beginning, a middle, and an end. The same is true for rituals, and the ending is just as important as all the other parts. In rituals you are working with powerful energies, and these need to be consciously dispersed, bidden farewell, and let go. Just as you would not leave a party before finding the host and hostess and thanking them, neither would you leave a ritual without the appropriate ending.

There are two aspects of ending rituals—the physical, material part, and the mental, emotional part. The latter is done first, and usually you meditate for a few minutes at the end of a ritual. This gives time and space for reflection, the acknowledgment of completion, and assessment of whether the intention was satisfied. It also gives a few moments of silence, which is how creation began and will undoubtedly end. It is also common to feel inspired and creative at this time, and whatever you do afterward will benefit from the quality of the ritual.

Clearing up all objects used is important too, especially if other people will use the same space. This decenters the energies, bringing the space back into mundane reality. The clearing up is still part of the ritual, albeit the last part, and is done thoroughly with conscious intent.

With group rituals it is traditional to feast together afterward, and share experiences. There is an intimacy to the group brought about by the ritual that united everyone's energies and aspirations. Enjoying a meal together, with a little wine perhaps,

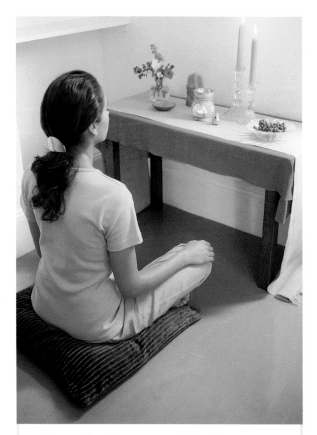

Concluding meditation
The meditation at the end of a ritual gives time and space for reflection, the acknowledgment of completion, and an assessment of how well the intention of the ritual was realized through the ritual ceremony.

provides relaxation after the accomplishment of the task, and makes a gentle transition from ritual to the everyday world. Sharing experiences with each other is also an informal way to learn and understand more about the ritual.

Bereavement and Letting Go Ritual

"The present life and all its experiences are fleeting; clinging to anything in this world is like chasing a rainbow. If we keep this in mind constantly we will not waste time on mundane pursuits, but spend it wisely."

KATHLEEN MCDONALD: *HOW TO MEDITATE*

DEATH IS A PART OF THE WHOLE LIFE PROCESS; it completes the circle started at conception. Without death, there could not be life. We know death is inevitable; however, we usually try to forget what we see as an unpleasant future event, considering death only when it touches someone we know.

Bereavement and grieving rituals help us to express whatever emotions we need to, and feelings can be more complex than just sadness at the death of a close friend or relative. Death can make us feel guilty, angry, even happy if the person we loved suffered a great deal before dying and death was a merciful release. However, we might feel it is wrong to associate death with anything other than grief.

Modern Western culture has lost many of its rituals, and death and bereavement rituals are no exception. We often don't express our feelings; instead we try to bottle them up inside. Repressed feelings have a habit of surfacing when we least expect them to, and often in another and unhealthy guise.

Traditional periods of mourning, symbolized by wearing black clothes, have been shortened to a couple of days' compassionate leave from our job. We are made to feel guilty if we haven't recovered after that. The wailing and weeping of other cultures is often considered excessive and exhibitionist, and, except for the funeral ceremony, there is little ritual around death. This makes it important to find, adapt, or make a bereavement ritual for yourself.

This ritual is also useful for the end of a pet's life, the "death" of a job, relationship, fertility on reaching menopause, and other life changes involving loss. Aromatics have always been used in death rituals in all cultures, and essential oils are invaluable, whether to honor the dead ritually by anointing, or to soothe and help let go of our feelings.

Lilies

Lilies are often associated with death, though the original pagan association was with virgin motherhood. Lily was the flower of Lilith, the Sumero-Babylonian Goddess of Creation, representing the virgin aspect of the Triple Goddess.

A Bereavement Ritual

The intent of this ritual is to honor the person, pet, job, relationship, or whatever or whoever has died. Choose an essential oil to banish negative energies, one to reflect the character of the deceased, and one to honor your own feelings. Light your burner with these three oils.

Meditate on impermanence, that the grief you now feel will pass, and that you too will die. Bring the deceased to mind, and recall shared moments. Think of the deceased fondly, and thank him or her for sharing time with you.

Visualize the person, situation, or other, with yourself enclosed in a circle of light—white, gold, or whatever color you resonate with at this time. Creatively imagine a farewell ceremony between you.

When it feels the right time to let go, visualize the circle dividing like a fertilized ovum, separating the two of you. Let the deceased go in peace, and send the person your blessing as his or her circle of light spins away through the universe.

Sit quietly with your feelings, and ask yourself if there is any emotion you need to express. You may want to cry, wail, shout, write, dance, play a drum, or light a fire. Give yourself permission to do the thing you need to do, as long as it does not involve hurting any living being. Either do it now, or resolve to do it soon.

Sit quietly for as long as you need. End the ritual by reflecting that you have honored the deceased and your own feelings. This ritual can be repeated if required; death and transition can affect us for longer than we think, or society finds acceptable.

Group Rituals

"An intimate and well-functioning ritual group can help each member deal with his or her psychic banishing, reprogramming, growth process and personal adjustments in a timely and extremely effective manner."

DENNY SARGENT: *GLOBAL RITUALISM*

SEVERAL OF THE RITUALS DESCRIBED IN THIS BOOK can be performed alone or in a group. They are all simple rituals—but powerful and effective—that give a taste of the ritual experience. You may wish to explore further, and a regular ritual group is helpful. Ritual is a huge and complex subject, and in a group each member can take turns to research a particular ritual, or culture's rituals, to share with the group.

This allows the group to benefit from each individual's knowledge. Sharing in this way is mutually enriching; not just in terms of acquiring knowledge but in terms of developing trust, goodwill, and respect for each other. Ritual often causes powerful feelings to arise as we connect with universal and natural energies. This can be overwhelming at times, and supporting each other facilitates the whole group's learning process.

All participants need to make a commitment to the group process, because intermittent attendance is unsettling and disrupts the energy flow. So it is sensible to keep your group numbers small, and to hold meetings perhaps once a month at the beginning. It is wiser not to overstretch yourselves and then give up. Initial excitement tends to wear off quickly, and you will soon see who has made a real commitment and who had just a passing interest. Keep your ritual group private and introduce others carefully. Many people mock, fear, or have an unhealthy interest in ritual, so secrecy is important, although you do not need to be obsessive about it. You should allow common sense to prevail.

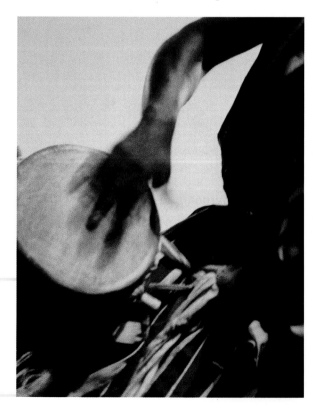

Drumming

This Moroccan drummer uses the power of rhythm and a regular beat to elevate his consciousness. This facilitates ritual working, and in group rituals helps everyone tune into the same wavelength.

Ritual for Group Harmony

This is a good ritual with which to start a group. The intention is to promote harmony between everyone, to learn how to perform a basic ritual, and to give a sense of purpose to your ritual work.

Start with a simple banishing such as washing your hands and removing your shoes before entering the room. Create your sacred space by sitting in a circle, holding hands meditating on the breath for five or ten minutes.

The group should then select a blend of essential oils that everyone likes, but don't let this degenerate into individual egos striving for supremacy. If things get complicated, select just one essential oil that symbolizes harmony for everyone.

Light the burner, and then each member in turn should perform a simple offering. This can be offering to the four directions, chanting, or reciting a prayer or poem while holding the burner, or a silent offering holding the burner aloft. Experimentation will produce variations. Support everyone's attempts; it may take time for certain people to feel comfortable trying out their offerings.

Inviting harmonious energies into your sacred space follows. This can be done with drumming, dancing, or chanting— whatever the group consensus is for this particular occasion.

The rhythm of your drumming or other activity brings everyone's energies onto the same wavelength. Hold in mind the intention of creating harmony between everyone. Don't try to intellectualize this process; just feel the energy.

Allow your sensitivity to the group energy to bring this to a close naturally. This works only if everyone is sensitive to everyone else; individual ego desires are out of place.

End your ritual by sitting in a circle holding hands and doing mindfulness meditation. Analyze your experiences afterward, but be joyful and playful, not critical. Share a meal together with some wine and organize what the group will do next time.

Personal Talisman or Amulet

"In this way amulets can be said to be solidified or personified synchronicity. From their discovery or creation to their use, they are part and parcel of tilting the plane of existence so that desired synchronicities will come the wearer's way."

DENNY SARGENT: *GLOBAL RITUALISM*

OBJECTS OF POWER, CALLED TALISMANS OR amulets, are used all over the world, as much in the modern West as in more traditional cultures. Sportsmen and -women often have a personal good-luck charm, and believe that it brings them winning luck, or, if the sport is dangerous, keeps them safe.

Religious people use many sacred objects as amulets. Christians, for example, may wear a cross or an image of Saint Christopher. Religious texts can be amulets, such as Tibetan Buddhist prayer flags, which are inscribed with sacred texts and mantras. These are strung from temples and trees; every time the wind moves them, the prayers are blown around as a blessing.

It is the belief in the efficacy of the object rather than any intrinsic quality that counts, though objects that have been used for a long time as amulets have a charged quality. If your culture has faith in a talisman, then you will have a strong unconscious link with the object, such as Native Americans have with their tribal totems.

Amulets bring good luck and repel bad luck. They can attract a lover, help conception, cure illness, and prevent accidents. Divination by runes, tarot cards, or the *I Ching* (an ancient Chinese oracle) are popular. Creating your own personal amulet with specific essential oils according to the occasion combines the power of faith in the talisman with the intrinsic qualities of the essential oils.

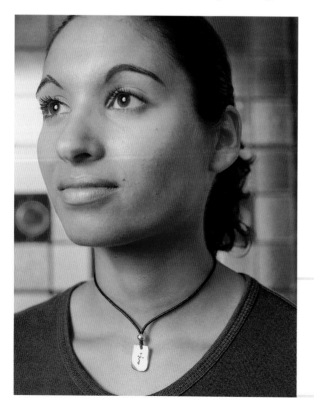

Objects of power

Many people wear amulets around their necks to bring good luck and repel bad luck. These can be personally charged with superstitious belief, or part of a religious tradition, such as the Christian cross, or Saint Christopher pendant.

An amulet with essential oils

An essential oil amulet is ritually anointed before the event you wish to influence. Meditating beforehand, burning the oil or blend you wish to use, will enhance the effect and also ensure that you have chosen the correct essential oils. Remember—it is your belief that your essential oil amulet will work that will charge its efficacy.

Anointing with essential oils must be done with care and firm intent. Certain essential oils are skin irritants, and unless you feel strongly drawn to one, they are best avoided. Some oils are safe to use directly on the skin, such as the floral oils, but after applying if you notice any irritation wash off immediately and apply some unperfumed skin cream. If in doubt, or if you are using potentially irritant oils, you can "anoint" your hair or clothing instead.

An amulet with essential oils for attracting a lover is always popular! Before going out to dance, for example, you would prepare yourself, starting with the bath ritual already described. Choose oils you find erotic and in the bath reflect on the reasons you wish to attract a lover. Choosing clothes, dressing, and applying makeup form your own personal ritual. But do not use perfume; your amulet of essential oils provides all the perfume you will need.

A powerful attraction blend is jasmine for confidence and erotic power, neroli for nervousness and soft femininity, and sandalwood to keep you grounded in the sexual chakra. You might like to wear just ylang ylang or rose on its own; only you know what works for you.

Stand in front of your mirror and look at yourself without judgment. Surface beauty is skin deep; it is

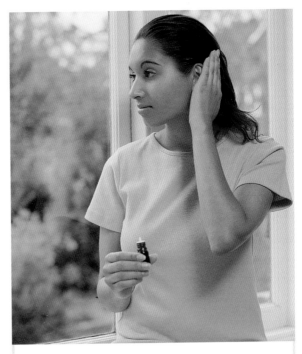

Anointing hair

If your essential oil amulet contains potentially skin-irritant essential oils, it is best not to apply this directly to the skin. A good alternative is to stroke the oils through your hair.

inner beauty that attracts, and belief in yourself that counts. We are loved for who we are, not what we look like, unless this is what we choose. Take up your oil or blend and apply a drop behind each ear, and on each wrist, or brush the oils through your hair and over your clothes. Trust they will attract a lover; if they don't do it tonight, then they will help to do it later. This is your personal essential oil amulet, and each time you wear it with conviction, you are creating the causes for the eventual fulfillment of your desire.

Bibliography

Ashcroft-Nowicki D., *First Steps in Ritual*, Thorsons, London, 1990

Barks C., *The Essential Rumi*, HarperCollins, London, 1995

Batchelor S., *The Awakening of the West*, HarperCollins, London, 1994

Bates B., *The Way of Wyrd*, Arrow Books, London, 1996

Battaglia S. & Kerr J., (eds), *Aromatherapy Today*, Vols 7, 11, 13, 1998–2000

Butler W., *Magic Its Ritual, Power & Purpose*, Aquarian Press, London, 1971

Culpeper, N., *Culpeper's Complete Herbal*, W. Foulsham & Co. Ltd., 1952

Dalai Lama, *A Policy of Kindness*, Snow Lion Publications, New York, 1990

Dalai Lama, *Kindness, Clarity & Insight*, Snow Lion Publications, New York, 1993

Dalai Lama, *Secular Meditation* (video), The Foundation for Universal Responsibility, Delhi, 1996

Davis P., *Aromatherapy: An A–Z*, C. W. Daniels, Saffron Walden, 1995

Fischer-Rizzi S., *Complete Aromatherapy Handbook*, Jain Publishers, New Delhi, 1998

Grieve M., *A Modern Herbal*, Harcourt, Brace & Company, New York, 1931

Lawless J., *The Encyclopedia of Essential Oils*, Element Books, Shaftesbury, 1992

McDonald K., *How to Meditate*, Wisdom Publications, Boston, 1984

Mailhebiau P., *Portraits in Oils*, C. W. Daniels, Saffron Walden, 1995

Maury M., *Marguerite Maury's Guide to Aromatherapy*, C. W. Daniels, Saffron Walden, 1989

Moncrieff R.W., *Odours*, 1970

Sargent D., *Global Ritualism*, Llewellyn Publications, Minnesota, 1994

Snelling J., *The Buddhist Handbook*, Rider, London, 1997

Tisserand R., *Aromatherapy for Everyone*, Penguin Books, London, 1988

Tisserand R., *The Art of Aromatherapy*, C. W. Daniels, Saffron Walden, 1987

Titmuss C., *The Power of Meditation*, Quarto Books, London, 1999

Worwood V., *Aromantics*, Pan Books, London, 1987

Useful Addresses

Essential Oils Suppliers

Absolute Essentials, Derrynaneal, Feakle, Co. Clare, Eire.
e-mail: absolute@esatclear.ie

Aroma Vera, 3384 South, Robertson Place, Los Angeles, CA 90034, USA

Essentially Oils, 8 Mount Farm, Junction Rd, Churchill, Chipping Norton,
Oxfordshire, OX7 6NP, UK. Tel: + 44 (0)1608 659544

Liberty Natural Products, 8120 SE Street, Portland 97215, USA.
Tel: (001) 800 289 8247. www.libertynatural.com

Neal's Yard U.S.A., 284 Connecticut Street, San Francisco, CA 94107, USA

Springfields Aromatherapy, Unit 2, 2 Anella Avenue, Castle Hill 2154,
Australia. International Tel: + 61 2 9894 9933

Verde Mail Order International, 3 Princes Close, Old Town, London, SW4
0LQ, UK. Tel: + 44 (0)207 720 1100

Meditation Centers

Gaia House, West Ogwell, Newton Abbot, Devon, TQ12 6EN, UK.
Tel: + 44 (0)1626 333613

Insight Meditation Society, 1230 Pleasant Street, Barre, MA 01005, USA.
Tel: (001) 978 355 4378.

Index